Life's Journey

*A Guide from Conception to Growing Up,
Growing Old, and Natural Death*

✛

Gerard M. Verschuuren

Life's Journey

*A Guide from Conception to
Growing Up, Growing Old,
and Natural Death*

Foreword by
Ronald S. Arellano, M.D.

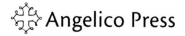 Angelico Press

First published
by Angelico Press 2016
© Gerard M. Verschuuren 2016

For information, address:
Angelico Press
4709 Briar Knoll Dr.
Kettering, OH 45429
angelicopress.com

978-1-62138-164-8 (pbk)
978-1-62138-165-5 (ebook)

NIHIL OBSTAT
Fr. Joseph M. Gile, S.T.D.
Censor Librorum, Diocese of Wichita, KS

IMPRIMATUR
Bishop Carl A. Kemme, D.D.
Bishop of Wichita, KS

Cover design: Michael Schrauzer

✝

Dedicated to my beloved deceased parents,
who enabled my life's journey

CONTENTS

Foreword

Dr. Verschuuren, an accomplished scientist, author, and speaker, has created a masterful work in his most recent book, titled *Life's Journey: A Guide from Conception to Natural Death.*

In this work, Dr. Verschuuren expertly explains the basic science of the physical body and its various growth and maturation processes from conception through death in very readable terms. He has organized each chapter into two parts: "The Biology Behind It," where Dr. Verschuuren the scientist eloquently carries the reader through the basic science of each stage of life. It is in these sections of each chapter that his exceptional gift of writing and explaining complex concepts in extremely readable prose shines through. For those readers who may feel intimated by scientific writing, rest assured that these sections are apt to captivate the scientific and non-scientific reader alike.

In the second part of each chapter, titled "Behind the Biological Facts," Dr. Verschuuren the philosopher and observer of human nature overlays the biological "facts" with well-reasoned concepts accessible to all of us that are not easily explained, and even rejected, by science, but that equally contribute to the human organism. For example, the discussion in Chapter 4 of rationality and morality is so intriguing and captivating that no reader of this book can fail to walk away feeling challenged to consider his or her own life, the factors that lead to our own decision-making, and the impact of these decisions on others.

Throughout his book, the author seems to challenge the reader with at least two overt questions: "what are we?" ("The biology behind it," that is), and "who are we?" ("The philosophy behind the facts"). In so doing, Dr. Verschuuren coherently and convincingly argues that we are more than just an assemblage of molecules. This, in turn, leads the reader to an equally important implicit question: "Is there purpose to who and what we are?"

In Chapter 6, Dr. Verschuuren touches on the last, very important question; and, without being pedantic, challenges the reader to consider the role of religion in the human condition, with what he explains as a "cosmic design." And while we as humans tend to think in the "here and now," Dr. Verschuuren points to an expanded version of this concept—that the "here and now" is really part of a journey, the continuation of which begins with the "tomb."

RONALD S. ARELLANO, M.D.
Massachusetts General Hospital
Associate Professor of Radiology,
Harvard Medical School

Acknowledgments

I wish to express my gratitude to those who steered and corrected me in the process of preparing this book. In particular, I want to mention Ronald Arellano, M.D. (Massachusetts General Hospital and Harvard University), Francisco Ayala (University of California at Irvine), Stephen Barr (University of Delaware), Paul Camarata, M.D. (University of Kansas School of Medicine), Peter Kreeft (Boston College), and also some great minds from my past in the Netherlands who helped to shape my mind before they passed away: the philosopher Cornelis van Peursen and the biologist Marius Jeuken, S.J., both of Leiden University; and the human biologist John Huizinga, M.D., of Utrecht University Medical School.

And—as with all my English books—I could not have written this book without the unwavering and loving support of my wife, Trudy. I also want to specifically mention the helpful advice of our granddaughter Chelsea Kelley, Graduate and Transfer Admissions Counselor at MCPHS University (Massachusetts College of Pharmacy and Health Sciences) in Boston, who helped me in polishing the text.

These and many others make me realize that originality often consists in the capacity to forget about one's own sources. Obviously, they are not responsible for the outcome—if any error remains, it is entirely my doing.

Preface

This book is about not only biology, but also about the Great Questions of Life and Death. Although there is a lot of science in this book, taking us through all the biological milestones of life's journey, it is also a critical and intellectual philosophical journey, starting in the world of science but ultimately in pursuit of the Great Questions that permeate the course of everyone's life throughout all of its stages.

This book describes the six main phases of life's journey in varying degrees of detail. Some of these stages you have already gone through yourself; others are still ahead of you. But no matter where you are at this point in your life, this journey is yours. You may not be able to retrace previous stages, but you are probably anxious to know what is ahead of you. And besides, you may have children or grandchildren who are going through earlier stages, or parents who are experiencing later stages. In all these situations, I think this book has something to offer you.

Each chapter discusses one specific stage of your life's journey. Every chapter begins with a biological description of that period in life, followed by a more philosophical reflection. One cannot be without the other. We need facts before we can reflect, but facts without reflection are meaningless.

The first section of each chapter ("The Biology Behind It") presents the most important and relevant scientific data marking the big milestones in every human life. It is like a handbook of what human beings go through in their life-cycle. In order to keep the book readable for the more general reader, no footnotes mentioning the sources of the data are included. Yet be assured that, being a scientist myself, I have tried to only select for inclusion information that is reliable and has been corroborated.

The second section of each chapter ("Behind the Biological Facts") offers a reflection on the scientific data presented in the pre-

3

Life's Journey

vious section. This places the "factual" information in a wider context. Sometimes these reflections are more philosophical in nature; sometimes they look at the scientific issue from a different perspective, or at least from a wider perspective, such as a moral or religious one. Sometimes they question extravagant claims.

I do not believe that we should always give biologists and physicists the last word. In this book they get the first word, as it were, and help set the right tone; but it is my strong conviction that there is more to life than what scientists tell us when they dish out their scientific facts. I tried not to be too much of a scientist for philosophical minds, or too much of a philosopher for scientific minds. I deeply believe that both have much to learn from each other.

1

From the Day of Conception

THE BIOLOGY BEHIND IT

"Where shall I begin?" asked the White Rabbit of the King in *Alice's Adventures in Wonderland.* "Begin at the beginning, and go on till you come to the end: then stop." That is good advice when talking about life's journey—begin at the beginning. Most likely, none of us has any conscious memories of the event that started our lives when a sperm cell penetrated an egg cell. We have no personal memories of what happened at that moment, but scientific research does provide us with some idea of it.

Interestingly enough, the philosopher Aristotle retained the view that the sperm just empowered the womb to provide the nutrients for the growth of a new person. This prolific "seed" was believed to bring into the womb a "living principle" that had the power to generate new life—the rest, and only the rest (namely, the nutrients), Aristotle thought, came from the mother's womb. It took a long time before biologists began to realize that—in addition to nutrients—the mother also provides another very essential element of the generation of new life, an egg cell.

The Origin of New Life

William Harvey (1578–1657), best known as the first scientist to discover that our blood supply is on the work of a closed, circulatory system, also seems to have reached a more accurate understanding of what happens during procreation when he said that new life comes forth from eggs. However, what he meant by "egg" was basically a food package—it could be an egg (as with chickens), but also menstrual blood (as with mammals), or even putrefied material (as with insects and worms).

5

Yet the search for eggs was on. In 1652, Johannes van Horne actually located them in what we call nowadays the ovaries of females, but then in 1672 Regnier de Graaf discovered that these "eggs," now called follicles, only contain fluid and actually burst open; what happened next remained unclear to him. It would take much longer before it was discovered that these follicles do contain an egg cell.

In the meantime, the Dutchman Antonie van Leeuwenhoek had turned attention from eggs to sperm again when he discovered with his microscope that sperm contains "small animals," as he described them—some kind of miniature organisms. By the 1690s, biologists such as Hartsoeker and Dalempatius were convinced that through their simple microscopes they could actually discern a miniscule human being inside each human sperm cell. So the battle was on between those claiming that the embryo comes from sperm, believed to be merely in search of food stored in the egg, and those believing that the embryo actually comes from the egg, which then only would need sperm for it to be activated.

Nowadays it has become common knowledge that the embryo cannot be found in sperm and cannot be found in the egg, as together they both contribute to the process of generation. Human beings carry 23 *pairs* of matching chromosomes—of which one is an unmatched pair of sex chromosomes in males (XY), but a "real" pair (XX) in females. For procreation it is necessary that males produce sperm cells with an unpaired half-set of 23 chromosomes and that females release egg cells, again with an unpaired half-set of 23 chromosomes. For males, starting in puberty, the production of sperm cells occurs continuously in the testes. For females, starting in puberty and ending during menopause, the formation of egg cells occurs in the ovaries, but the release of one of these only happens once in a cycle of 28 days, in a process called ovulation; hormones such as estradiol and progesterone are an important part of this menstrual cycle (more on this later).

Nowadays, science has given us a better understanding of what happens when a sperm cell penetrates an egg cell. When a sperm cell, containing only one set of 23 chromosomes, and an egg cell, containing also a single set of 23 chromosomes, come together, they fuse their chromosomes and start a new organism with 23 *pairs* of chromosomes again. So what happens at conception is that father and mother each contribute only a half set of their chromosomes, one of each pair, so their child ends up again with 23 pairs. Depending on whether the father passed on his X- or his Y-chromosome, the child will be male (XY) or female (XX). The child may look more like the father or more like the mother, yet they both contributed the same amount of chromosomes.

Chromosomes and Genes

What do these chromosomes carry? The simplest answer is "genes." Since all genes are located in these chromosomes, they come in pairs as well. Let us briefly discuss first what a gene is.

Since the discovery of DNA, the boundaries of a gene have become rather fuzzy, but a classical definition has it that a gene is a unit of heredity that regulates a specific trait, feature, or characteristic of an organism: there are genes that are thought to regulate our blood types, our eye colors, and so forth. Each gene can carry several variants, called *alleles*. Since genes come in pairs, they can carry either two different alleles or two of the same allele. It is the different alleles of a gene that cause genetic differences between individuals. In short, all humans have in essence the same genes, but not the same alleles—and it seems that differences in alleles make them different from each other.

Just what do these genes cause? How do they operate? What does it mean when someone says there is "a gene for…"? Here is a brief explanation. Most genes create specific enzymes, or other proteins. When a gene carries an abnormal allele, it may produce a non-functional protein that cannot do its normal work.

Some diseases can be traced back to one specific gene that carries one or two abnormal alleles. Although such *mono*-factorial cases are rather rare, they do exist. Simple yet sometimes serious genetic disorders such as sickle cell anemia do follow the mono-factorial, one-step scenario. Sickle-cell anemia is a genetic blood disorder characterized by red blood cells that assume an abnormal, rigid sickle shape, which can cause various complications, such as anemia. The sickling occurs because of an abnormal allele for the formation of the oxygen-carrying protein hemoglobin in red blood cells.

This is just a simple case of how a gene works—one gene can directly lead to one specific disease if it carries the abnormal allele. And there are a few more examples, such as muscular dystrophy, Huntington's disease and Tay-Sachs disease—the latter two of which both cause progressive mental deterioration—and a common form of dwarfism called achondroplasia. A more widely known example is phenylketonuria; in this case, there is one gene that produces a certain enzyme called *phenylalanine hydroxylase*. This gene can also harbor mutated alleles that produce a non-functional enzyme, which then may cause mental retardation, seizures, and other serious medical problems if the patient does not follow a strict phenylalanine-free diet. What all these diseases have in common is that they follow a simplified formula: one gene can lead to one specific disease if it carries one or sometimes two versions of the wrong allele; if one version is enough to cause the disease, it is called *dominant*.

Most cases, however, do not belong to this category. The vast majority of human diseases and other genetic traits are multi-factorial: they are influenced by many genes interacting with one another. Besides, they are also affected by a vast array of signals from the environment of each cell (nutrient supply, hormones, electrical signals from other cells, etc.)—all of which together reflect the external world of the organism as a whole (upbringing, learning, experience, culture, religion). Thus, the same mutation in a specific gene may produce very different results, depending on their surrounding background as well as on their genetic background (that is, all other interacting genes combined), as each human being has a background that is unique. No two persons are completely identical—not even when their genes carry the same alleles, as is typically the case with identical twins. Identical twins do not even have identical fingerprints. We have discovered that their DNA is not exactly the same either, especially in its non-coding parts. In short, even "identical" twins are not fully identical.

A decade ago, the general estimate for the number of human genes was thought to be well over 100,000, but turned out to be around 22,500—which is only a bit more than the 19,735 genes of a tiny roundworm. And humans have only 300 genes not also found in mice. No wonder that Craig Venter, the president of Celera, a bio-corporation, said of this surprising finding: "This tells me genes cannot possibly explain all of what makes us what we are." At least, there is a first indication here that genes are not as almighty as some would have us believe.

DNA, the Language of Genes

What is it that these genes carry? The simplest answer is DNA. A molecule of DNA (Deoxyribo-Nucleic Acid) is composed of building blocks called *nucleotides*, each of which is itself composed of a five-carbon sugar bonded to a phosphate group and a nitrogenous base.

For the hungry minds among you, the following will be of interest (otherwise, you may skip this section). There are four kinds of nucleotides in DNA, which differ from one another in their nitrogenous bases: adenine (A) and guanine (G) are double-ring structures, whereas cytosine (C) and thymine (T) are single-ring structures. In a DNA molecule the nucleotides are arranged in sequence, held together by covalent bonds between the sugar of one nucleotide and the phosphate group of the next nucleotide beyond it; the nitrogenous bases are arranged as side groups off the chains. DNA molecules ordinarily exist as double-chain structures—comparable to a zipper—with the two chains held together by hydrogen bonds between their nitrogenous bases; such bonding can occur only between C and G (C-G bonds) or between T and A (T-A bonds). Finally, the ladder-like double-chain molecule is coiled into a double helix.

For a while, geneticists held on to what they literally called their "central dogma," which claims that "DNA makes RNA makes protein"—that is, a one-directional causal flow, with one item of code, a gene, ultimately making one item of substance, a protein (proteins include also enzymes). So it appears that the DNA of a gene forms a sequence of amino acids, and all these proteins together are responsible for the human body. Since there are four different nucleotides (A, C, G, and T) and twenty different amino acids, the coding unit of DNA—a *codon*—must be three nucleotides long, which makes for 64 possible combinations (4^3) and thus leaves room for synonyms. The codons GCA, GCC, GCG, and GCU, for example, all specify the same amino acid, alanine.

DNA acts as a template for synthesis of messenger RNA (mRNA), which in turn determines the order of amino acids in enzymes and other proteins. The two strands of a DNA molecule in the cell nucleus first un-couple so that one of the two strands can act as a template for synthesis of a complementary string of mRNA; mRNA leaves the nucleus and goes to the cytoplasm, where it complexes with ribosomes; tRNA carries one specific amino acid to mRNA at a time; tRNA couples briefly with mRNA on a ribosome; the ribosome moves along on mRNA, adding amino acids to the growing polypeptide chain, which finally results in a protein; tRNA moves off to pick up a new amino acid.

However, our view of this process has dramatically changed recently. First of all, some DNA sections, known as *introns*, get initially transcribed into mRNA but are then removed from the end-product by a process called splicing. Due to alternative splicing, a single gene may code for several different proteins. This phenomenon would partially explain why the number of genes can be much lower than was initially expected.

Second, genes can be overlapping; about 9% of human protein-coding genes overlap another such gene. Sometimes the overlaps are partial, but in other cases small protein-coding genes are fully embedded within much larger genes (e.g., blood-clotting factor VIII)—so that they are essentially genes-within-genes. In this way, a certain DNA sequence may make a contribution to the function of several gene products. In other cases, some DNA sequences do double-duty, encoding one protein when read along one strand and a second protein when read in the opposite direction along the other strand.

Third, it was discovered that protein-coding regions of genes can be interrupted by DNA segments that play more of a regulatory role. They do so by producing activator and repressor proteins that respectively activate or repress the activity of a "regular" gene. Some of these regulatory genes are very short and produce not proteins, but short strands of mRNA capable of blocking the mRNA of a regular gene from creating its protein; these genes are called micro-RNA genes.

Fourth, some genes have lost their functionality—they are called pseudo-genes. These genes resemble a regular DNA-packet of a functional gene, but they have been affected by one or more glitches that change their script into "nonsense." They were once functional genes but have since lost their protein-coding ability—and thus, presumably, their biological function. When comparing humans and chimpanzees, we do find genes that are functional in one species but not in another, and are thus nominally pseudo-genes. A striking example is the gene for a jaw-muscle protein (*MYH16*), which has become a pseudo-gene in humans, but is still successfully codes for the development of strong jaw muscles in other primates. Another example is the DNA sequence for an enzyme that produces ascorbic acid, or vitamin C, in most animals. Many primates, including humans, have a defect in this DNA code, so they must acquire vitamin C through food—yet they hold on to this pseudo-gene.

And then there has been a fifth important development. Genes may be separated by long stretches of DNA that do not seem to be doing much at all—that is why they are often called "junk DNA," in spite of the fact that it would be much safer to speak here of "non-coding," "neutral," or "silent" DNA. Some of this "non-coding" DNA is repetitive DNA, often replicated from regular, coding DNA, and perhaps a rich source from which potentially useful new genes can emerge during evolution. Regarding simple genetic inheritance, the story is getting more and more complicated.

Yet since the ultimate goal of most scientists seems to be an explanation of life in terms of DNA, the "secret of life" is supposed to reside in DNA. On this view, all that counts is DNA; so with the *Human Genome Project* finished, we are supposed to know all there is to know about human beings. Because of all these new discoveries, many people now think that it is DNA that holds the script for a person's entire life, and accordingly they seek to determine their "personal genomics." No wonder DNA pioneer Sidney Brenner claimed not too long ago that he could compute an entire organism if he were given its DNA sequence and a sufficiently large computer. DNA seems to have become the definitive controlling agency behind each human life. We will see if this is in fact the case.

Twins, Triplets...

Now we shall consider again the role of sperm cells and egg cells. The release of an egg cell, with its own DNA, by one of the two ovaries in a woman's body is regulated by a complex network of hormones. As Sherman J. Silber, M.D., of St. Luke's Hospital in St. Louis, explains, women are born with all the eggs they are ever going to have; they do not make any additional eggs during their lifetime. They are born with approximately 2,000,000 eggs in their ovaries, but about 11,000 of them die every month prior to puberty. At the onset of puberty, the average woman will have some 300,000 to 400,000 eggs left. An average of 1,000 will die every month, and each month only one of those thousand will make it to ovulation.

Each egg cell is enclosed within a resting follicle, which contains, in addition to the developing egg cell, the support cells that surround and nourish it. Most of the 400,000 follicles in a woman's ovaries are dormant, but out of that primordial pool some will begin to develop each day. The younger the woman and the larger the total number of eggs in her ovaries, the greater the number of eggs in any given month, or on any given day, that will leave their resting stage and develop into ripe follicles.

Every day, thirty or so previously dormant eggs emerge by some still unknown signal into the three-month process of ripening, beginning their eighty-five days of development with the goal of eventually trying to ovulate. So at any time in the ovaries, there are early-stage, resting follicles; there are somewhat larger follicles; others are beginning to form a fluid-filled space; and there are ripe follicles. In the middle of the menstrual cycle, on day fourteen, there is normally one dominant follicle, ready for ovulation. Every month, only one—out of the 1,000 that "tried"—will ever make it.

How is it regulated that each month only *one* of these ripe follicles is destined to ovulate, while all the others will die? Dr. Silber again: During the first seventy days of its development, a follicle is completely independent of any hormonal influence; even the presence of a follicle-stimulating-hormone (FSH) and the monthly hormonal cycle have no influence yet. But once the follicles have ripened, they begin to become sensitive to stimulation by FSH from the pituitary gland. As these ripe follicles grow in response to FSH, the dominant one responds best to this stimulus and starts secreting estrogen and inhibin-B; these two hormones in turn suppress the pituitary secretion of FSH. As a consequence, the other ripe follicles face a decline in FSH and will rapidly die and disappear for lack of FSH.

So there is actually a "competitive struggle" taking place between all of these approximately thirty ripened follicles in order to determine which one will become the dominant follicle and ovulate on day fourteen. The follicle that is most sensitive to FSH in the first few days of the cycle becomes even more sensitized to FSH, and thus gains the lead over all the other follicles. The dominant follicle will never relinquish its lead, because it requires less FSH than the others to get the same degree of stimulation. Once the estrogen production exponentially peaks—around day twelve or thirteen—it stimulates a dramatic rise in another hormone from the pituitary gland, the luteinizing hormone (LH). It is this rise in LH that prepares the one remaining follicle for the process known as ovulation. In response to the surge in LH, the follicle enlarges rapidly. About 24 to 36 hours after the LH surge, the follicle ruptures and releases the egg cell.

This explains why only *one* egg cell typically leaves the ovary each month. However, in the rather unlikely event that *two* cells happen to both reach full maturity at around the same time, then both egg cells may be released, ready for fertilization, before the signal is sent for the other eggs to stop maturation and die. With *two* eggs ready for fertilization, they may both end up being fertilized, but if so, always by two different sperm cells. When this happens, the mother is pregnant with two human beings—we call them twins, more specifically dizygotic or non-identical twins. They can be of the same sex or of different sex. Since they do not have the same DNA, these twins are basically related to each other like regular brothers ("fraternal twins"), regular sisters ("sororal twins"), or a brother and a sister.

The reason why two (or even more) follicles ovulate at the same time is not fully understood. It may result from a genetic tendency, for women who have a family history of non-identical twins have a higher chance of bearing non-identical twins themselves, probably because there is a genetically linked tendency to hyper-ovulate.

Other factors that increase the odds of having non-identical twins include maternal age and the use of fertility drugs and other fertility treatments, as well as nutrition. Nutrition, for instance, might explain why members of the Yoruba tribe in Nigeria have the highest rate of twinning in the world, at 45–50 non-identical twin sets per 1,000 live births, possibly because of high consumption of a specific type of yam that contains a natural phyto-estrogen; this may stimulate the ovaries to release an egg from each side. It has also been suggested that IGF (insulin-like growth factor) increases the chance of non-identical twins; this may be connected to dairy products, especially in areas where growth hormones are given to cattle.

Then there are fertility treatments, which might explain why the twin birth rate in the United States has risen from 18.9 to 33.3 per 1,000 births. The same holds for the birth of triplets, quadruplets, and so forth. However, due to the limited size of the mother's womb, multiple pregnancies are much less likely to carry to full term than single births, with twin pregnancies lasting only 37 weeks on average (3 weeks under full term).

Unlike fraternal twins, identical twins arise from one single egg cell fertilized by one single sperm cell, and are therefore called monozygotic. As a result, their DNA is identical—except for mutations that may occur later on during their development (see Chapter 6). Obviously, they are almost always of the same sex, unless mutation interferes during development. Identical twins result when, very early in the developmental process, the growing embryo divides into two separate embryos. Spontaneous division of the zygote into two embryos is not considered to be a hereditary trait, but rather a spontaneous or random event—or at least an event not caused by any specific known cause. It happens at a rate of about 3 in every 1,000 deliveries worldwide and is evenly distributed in all populations around the world.

The timing of this separation has quite an impact on the further course of the pregnancy. If the separation happens during the first four days, both embryos have their own outer membrane (chorion), their own inner membrane filled with amniotic fluid, and their own placenta. If the separation happens during the next four days, they do share their chorion and placenta, but still have their own amniotic sacs. If the split is even later, then they share their placenta, chorion, as well as amniotic sac.

Much more unusual are cases of conjoined twins—previously called "Siamese" twins. They occur very infrequently, only 1 in 100,000 births, with an overall survival rate of approximately 25%. They are certainly considered "twins," which simply means two individuals. There are two contradictory explanations as to their origin. The traditional theory held that the fertilized egg at some stage of division *splits*, but only partially. The theory more widely accepted today assumes that the fertilized egg completely separates, but then stem cells in their search for similar cells find like-stem cells on the other twin and *fuse* the twins together.

Whatever their origin is, surgical separation of conjoined twins is not always advised—the quality of life of twins who remain conjoined is higher than is commonly assumed. Yet, separation is possible, although the surgery ranges from relatively simple to extremely complex. Former Surgeon General C. Everett Koop did groundbreaking work on surgery for conjoined twins while still the surgeon-in-chief at the Children's Hospital of Philadelphia. One of the main problems was that some conjoined twins would often bleed to death during surgery. In 1987, Dr. Ben Carson operated on the Binder twins by putting them in hypothermic arrest during surgery; as he wrote later, "lo and behold, it worked."

BEHIND THE BIOLOGICAL FACTS

It is time now to go behind the biological scenes and ask some pertinent and penetrating questions. The previous section may have created the impression that our life is wholly based on biological facts. Don't we all swear by the facts? Well, we should find out first what "facts" really are.

What Are the Facts?

When biologists say "the facts tell us…," they often think the discussion is closed, but "in fact" the discussion has just begun. It is not so obvious what the facts are. Francis Crick, one of the two co-discoverers of DNA, once said, "A theory that fits all the facts is bound to

15

be wrong, as some of the facts will be wrong." How could he say such a thing? How can facts be wrong? Are they not a matter of fact? Crick is right: facts are not the rock-solid realities most people think they are. What is "out there" is not an assortment of rock-solid facts, but rather a collection of things and events; facts are merely our *interpretations* of the things and events we see around us—they are our way of making them intelligible for us. Things and events may be the physical parts of our world, perhaps even rock-solid, but facts are mental creations—the interpretations of things and events in our minds. Facts are *about* something "rock-solid," about something beyond our control; but they are not "rock-solid" themselves, since they have a man-made dimension, dependent on human interpretation.

In observation, the observer is both a passive spectator and an active creator at the same time. We look at things as spectators, and then change them into facts as creators. We do not "have" observations, as we have sensory experiences; we "make" observations. Philosophical giants such as Aristotle and St. Thomas Aquinas would put it this way: All we know about the world comes through our senses, but is then processed by the intellect, which extracts from sensory experiences that which is intelligible. It is *facts*, produced by the intellect, that make things and events intelligible.

That is the reason why a camera, for instance, cannot capture facts—all it can capture is things and events. Take a surveillance camera; it "observes" everything because it does not know *what* to observe. That is why cameras cannot replace scientists—they may help them in their work, but cannot perform it for them. The problem with pictures is that they do not show us facts until we give some interpretation to the things and events we see in the picture. The same goes for books: they provide lots of information for "bookworms," but to real worms they have only paper to offer.

Here is a simple example of what this entails as far as facts are concerned. The more interpretation we inject into facts, the more information we can provide, but then we also increase what must be proven. By describing certain movements taking place in the sky as "moving spots" we convey information that is "empty" but "safe." By calling them "flying birds," however, we convey more information—and thus may need to come up with more evidence to support our claim. When we say instead, "Those are migrating geese," we inflate our claim even further, thus making this factual statement still more vulnerable to falsification. So what is the "real" fact here, one may ask—is it moving spots or flying birds or migrating geese or perhaps none of these? Only further investigation can show us the right interpretation of those perceived movements.

So far we have discussed one side of the coin: since facts are partly man-made, they often must to be revised. Many facts I learned in college while earning my degree in human biology and human genetics are now considered obsolete, and this may well happen again and again. So do not take the biological facts reported in this book as the final truth. It has even been claimed that more than half of recent biomedical findings cannot be reproduced. Facts are not as rock-solid as some would like them to be. You cannot take them at face value. Crick was right. And so was Spinoza when he said: "If facts conflict with a theory, either the theory must be changed or the facts."

But there is another side to the coin. Since facts are partly man-made, there can be many ways of looking at things—which makes for various sorts of facts. Facts are always interpreted from a specific perspective; and, since there are many more perspectives than what science tries to capture with its barometers, thermometers, and spectrometers, science does not provide us the only window on the world; there are many other windows, views, vistas.

Reality is like a jewel with many facets, and can be looked at from various angles, with different eyes, so to speak. Just as the physical eye sees colors in nature, so the "artistic eye" sees beauty in nature, the "rational eye" truths and untruths, the "moral eye" rights and wrongs, and the "religious eye" a divine dimension in life. All these "eyes" are in search of reality, but each one "sees" a different aspect of it—and therefore each one finds different "facts."

The physical or biological eye sees every beginning of new life as a fertilization process—a product of *procreation*. The "religious eye," on the other hand, sees it as a gift from Heaven—a product of *creation*. These two perspectives may be different, but are certainly not contradictory, as they can both be true and can equally qualify as "facts." In other words, a fertilized egg cell is the *beginning* of a human life, but it is not its *origin*. The origin of every human life is God, for God is the one about whom Genesis 1:1 says, "In the beginning, God created Heaven and Earth." It is in God that we live, move, and have our being. To put it differently: *In* the beginning of one's life is God, but *at* the beginning of one's life is a fertilized egg cell. Creation is something "in the beginning"—which makes it possible for each individual life to start "at the beginning." Each one of us came to this world *from* God, but *through* our parents.

The fact that God is the origin of all human life is as much "fact" as the fact that all human life comes from fertilized egg cells. All facts have a man-made component, seen from a specific perspective. By comparison, if you walk around a statue, what you see from the front is different than what you see from the back; yet both views are valid. Some facts—especially some scientific ones—come with an enormous baggage of background information and supporting observation techniques (without those, there would be no discovery of the Higgs boson, for instance); so do some religious facts. In other words, there are no "bare" facts—neither in science nor in religion.

Do not take this discussion the wrong way—it does not imply that facts are just mental creations, residing only in our minds. On the contrary, facts refer to things and events that have an existence independent of us, outside our minds. There is an objective order of things that we try to capture with our facts.

Is DNA the Secret of Life?

The previous section might suggest that the "secret" behind the development of a fertilized egg cell is located in the DNA coming from a sperm cell and an egg cell. Everything seems to start with, and as, DNA. No wonder this has led some to believe that our destiny is no longer written in the stars but in the genes.

Yet before endorsing this new mantra, we should pose the following question: How powerful is DNA really? Is it truly as powerful as some geneticists seem to suggest it is? Does the "secret of life" really reside in DNA? Is our destiny etched in DNA? Is DNA all there is and all that matters in the course of a human life? In response to these questions, it is necessary to debunk this widespread myth of DNA.

First of all, DNA can never do anything on its own. It is not even capable, as many still believe, of self-replication—making copies of itself on its own—for DNA copies are manufactured out of small molecular bits and pieces by the use of an elaborate cell machinery that is made up of proteins. If DNA is put in the presence of all the pieces that will be assembled into new DNA, but without any protein machinery, nothing happens. It is actually the surrounding cellular machinery that makes sure that old DNA strands are replicated into new strands. This process is analogous to the production of copies of a document by an office copying-machine—a process that would never be described as "self-replication." Think of viruses, which are essentially pure DNA or RNA; their DNA or RNA cannot do anything until they penetrate, like a Trojan horse, the interior of a living cell. So we have a chicken-and-egg problem here: DNA requires proteins, and proteins require DNA.

Second, DNA on its own does not produce anything, not even proteins. The role of DNA is to provide a specification as to how amino acids are to be strung together into proteins by some synthetic machinery; but this string of amino acids is not initially a protein. To become a protein with physiological and structural properties and functions, it must be folded into a three-dimensional configuration that is only partly based on its amino-acid sequence, but is also determined by the cellular environment and by special processing proteins.

Insulin for diabetics is a case in point. Recently, the DNA coding sequence for human insulin has been inserted into bacteria, which are then grown in large fermenters until a protein with the amino-acid sequence of human insulin can be extracted. But amino-acid sequence does not determine the shape of a protein. The first proteins harvested through this process did have the correct sequence, but were physiologically inactive. The bacterial cell had folded the protein incorrectly. Somehow the DNA does not itself "know" how to fold a protein so as to make it work. This problem may surface more often than was initially thought. Amyloids, for instance, are insoluble protein aggregates that arise from improperly folded polypeptides naturally present in the body. These mis-folded structures may even play a role in various neurodegenerative disorders, including Alzheimer's disease.

Third, the proteins that DNA produces do not only require a special folding process—it seems they may also need the presence of additional, non-protein factors that are not under direct DNA control, but come from the environment. Many proteins, especially those with enzymatic activity, need "helper molecules" to perform their biological function. These factors can be loosely-bound coenzymes, or tightly-bound prosthetic groups.

The enzymes alcohol dehydrogenase and DNA polymerase, for instance, require the presence of zinc as a cofactor for them to work. The hemoglobin protein in red blood cells, to take another example, requires the presence of a prosthetic heme group that contains iron in its center. The most common cofactors are metal ions such as iron, zinc, and copper; other cofactors are vitamins (vitamin C) or are made from vitamins (as in the case of B-vitamins). Without these cofactors, many DNA products cannot function properly; so it must be concluded that DNA by itself only delivers an incomplete product.

Fourth, if human beings were really nothing more than DNA, then it must have been the very DNA of the two scientists who discovered DNA, Watson and Crick, that discovered DNA. Think about this statement for a moment—DNA being discovered by DNA. If Watson and Crick were really nothing but DNA, then Watson's and Crick's DNA must have discovered itself. That would be like the magic of a projector projecting itself or a copy machine copying itself. However, we all know too well that we cannot pull ourselves up by our own bootstraps. DNA was discovered by Watson and Crick, not by their DNA.

Fifth, if we were nothing but DNA, this very statement—claiming that we are nothing but DNA—would not be worth more than its molecular origin, and neither would those who make such a statement. Claims like these defeat and destroy themselves. They cut off the very branch on which the person who utters them sits. If we want to accept the reliability of our biological knowledge regarding DNA, we cannot conclude at the same time that all human knowledge is just a product of DNA. In other words, those who make such claims must be more than just the DNA they carry. Therefore, we are always more than our DNA code. Even if you have an identical twin, with the same genetic code, you are still you, never him or her.

Sixth, there is the problem as to where our DNA comes from. Certainly, it comes from our parents, and they in turn received it from their parents. But that is not what I mean. Where did it ultimately come from? Most people would say it came from the animal world through a process of evolution based on natural selection. This is not the place to go into the discussion of whether this is true, or whether it is even possible (I have done so in other books). But even if it is true, the next question would be: How can DNA have the capacity to act as a "coding" language? Where does that capability ultimately come from?

The only feasible answer seems to be that this universe was created with an underlying *cosmic design* that regulates what is, and what is not, possible in this world. All the laws of nature are part of this cosmic design. The chemical element carbon (C), for instance, has the "built-in" ability to form very long chains of interconnecting C-C bonds; this property allows carbon to form an almost infinite number of compounds. That is the reason why the entire organic chemistry is carbon-based, making carbon the "favorite" building block of the living world on Planet Earth. When a die constantly throws a six, one would consider it loaded. Well, our world seems to be "loaded" too—loaded with cosmic design by the Creator of the universe. So it should not be surprising that carbon is an essential part of DNA as well—such is the way our world was designed in God's Mind.

There is a compelling case that the above considerations have taken DNA off its acclaimed pedestal. The inevitable outcome seems to be that DNA is not so much the "secret of life"—as so many claim—but rather the reverse, that life is the "secret of DNA." Ironically, the American molecular biologist Walter Gilbert had the audacity to declare that "when we have the complete sequence of the human genome we will know what it is to be human." That is at best professional—in fact unprofessional and unscientific—arrogance. Albert Einstein was probably right when he said, "the man of science is a poor philosopher" (although Einstein was a great exception himself).

Those who say "it's all about the DNA" belong to the same category of people as those who shout "it's all about money," "it's all about sex," or "it's all about politics." Those who thus narrow their outlook fail to realize that there is so much more to life. Such seemingly broad-minded slogans are actually narrow-minded ideologies which easily contradict each other. Fortunately most of us know how to take such expressions, as long as we do not take them literally.

As discussed earlier, even if we admitted that DNA is the basis of life, we would still need to acknowledge that this "fact" only represents a very limited perspective. There are many more valid perspectives on life, including religious perspectives. The fact that we came to be *through* DNA does not rule out that we ultimately came here *from* God. Put in a simple analogy: When someone receives an organ transplant, it comes through the hands of a surgeon, but the organ comes ultimately from a donor.

Can Things Go Wrong?

Can things go wrong when an egg cell and a sperm cell come together? The answer to this question is partially yes and partially no. Let us start with the positive dimension of the answer.

Human beings have two sets of 23 chromosomes, but during the production of sperm cells and egg cells, all pairs are split in half so the new cells have only one set of 23 chromosomes each. However, if the chromosome pairs *fail* to separate properly during cell division, the egg cell or sperm cell may end up with an extra copy of one of the chromosomes, giving the resulting embryo three copies instead of two (*trisomy*). Obviously, they may also end up with a missing copy (*monosomy*), but that is rather unusual.

What causes chromosomes to split improperly is not well understood. In general, this may become more likely with increasing age of the mother. It can happen to any of the 23 chromosomes; in most cases it leads to an early miscarriage. Estimates are that more than 50% of abortions occurring spontaneously in the first trimester of pregnancy are caused by chromosomal aberrations. However, some triple-state chromosomes do allow the organism to survive after birth. It may give rise to a handicap, but many of these people are able to live a happy and healthy life despite the challenge.

Some chromosomes—numbered or labeled as 21, 18, 13, X, and Y—are seen in live-born children as full trisomies, while trisomies of the chromosomes 15, 16, and 22 are often seen in miscarriages. The other chromosomes—1 to 12, 14, 17, 19, and 20—are almost never seen as full trisomies. Let us discuss in more detail the most common types of trisomy that survive to birth.

Trisomy 21, or Down syndrome, is the most common chromosome abnormality in humans. It is typically associated with some delay in cognitive ability and physical growth, and a particular set of facial characteristics. In spite of the fact that the average IQ of young adults with Down syndrome is lower than that of children without the condition, many children with Down syndrome do graduate from high school and are able to do paid work, and some go on to post-secondary education as well. Education and proper care have been shown to improve the quality of their lives significantly. And they certainly have a magnetic personality.

After Down syndrome, trisomy 18, or Edwards syndrome, is the second most common form of trisomy that carries to term. It occurs in around 1 in 6,000 live births, and around 80% of those affected are female. The majority of them die before birth. This syndrome's very low rate of survival is due to the concomitant heart abnormalities, kidney malformations, and other internal-organ disorders. About 8% of these infants survive longer than one year. Although women in their 20's and early 30's may conceive babies with this syndrome, the risk of doing so increases with a woman's age.

Trisomy 13, or Patau syndrome, causes infants to have difficulty surviving the first few days or weeks due to severe neurological problems or complex heart defects. Treatment focuses on the particular physical problems with which each child is born. Surgery may be necessary to repair heart defects or cleft lip and cleft palate. Physical, occupational, and speech therapy will help individuals with this syndrome reach their full developmental potential.

Trisomy XXY, or Klinefelter syndrome, is a condition in which an XY-person has an extra X-chromosome. Since these individuals do have a Y-chromosome, they will develop the male sexuality and are therefore usually referred to as "XXY Males." This form of trisomy occurs in roughly 1:500 to 1:1000 live male births, but many of these people may not show any symptoms. The physical traits of the syndrome, including reduced strength and reduced fertility, may only become more apparent after the onset of puberty, if at all.

Trisomy XXX, or Triple-X syndrome, causes a female to have an extra X chromosome in each of her cells. Because the vast majority of Triple-X females are never diagnosed, it may be very difficult to make generalizations about the effects of this syndrome. The reason why extra X-chromosomes have hardly any effect is that in female cells only one X-chromosome is active at any time, whereas any additional X-chromosomes are kept deactivated and remain condensed into so-called Barr-bodies.

The mechanism of deactivating additional X-chromosomes is not fully understood. It is somehow regulated by a gene on the X-chromosome called XIST. When this gene comes to expression, it produces a large non-coding RNA molecule that "silences" the X-chromosome from which it is transcribed by coating it with RNA molecules so it becomes inactive. It has been found that artificially placing and expressing the XIST gene on another chromosome leads to silencing of that chromosome as well. This has given researchers the hope that someday they might be able to also "silence" other redundant chromosomes in trisomy cases such as Down syndrome.

And then there is monosomy XO, or Turner syndrome. It is in a sense the opposite of trisomy—instead of three chromosomes, there is only one, with the second one missing (O). In 75% of the cases, the X-chromosome comes from the mother; the father does contribute an X-chromosome. Girls with Turner syndrome typically have dysfunctional ovaries, which results in sterility and having no menstrual cycle. Often there are also health concerns, such as congenital heart disease, reduced hormone secretion by the thyroid, diabetes, vision problems, hearing problems, and many autoimmune diseases. Hormone treatments are possible, though. It has been found that providing very low doses of estrogen to girls with Turner syndrome, as well as growth hormone, years before the onset of puberty increases their height and offers a wealth of other benefits.

A complication in the diagnosis of trisomy cases is that the third chromosome may not be a complete chromosome copy but only a partial one. In trisomy 9p, for instance, the third copy only consists of a portion of the short arm of chromosome 9. On the one hand, virtually all individuals with Trisomy 9p are affected by some mental retardation and distinctive malformations of the skull and facial region. On the other hand, trisomy 9p is one of the most frequent anomalies that has a high survival rate.

It should be noted, though, that all the trisomies mentioned so far may also develop *after* conception, during the production of new body cells, so they may only show up in a particular cell line. In such cases, only some of the body's cells have an extra (or missing) chromosome copy, resulting in a mixed population of cells with a differing number of chromosomes. Such cases are sometimes called *mosaic* syndromes. Very often the mosaic version of trisomy results in a very mild range of physical abnormalities and developmental delay compared to full-trisomy cases.

So as to the original question of whether things can go wrong at conception, the answer is "yes." But let us not forget that there is no "perfect" genome. Everybody has genetic flaws. It just depends on how such flaws become manifest in one's life. If you are looking for something wrong, you will certainly find it. In that sense, the answer is "yes"—things can go wrong.

However, seen in a different context, the answer could also be a cautious *no*. When we say that "things went wrong," we tend to think the result was a failure—and that could be a dangerous implication. Genes do not determine whether we are a failure or not; they are like a hand of cards we are dealt, but we can play them differently. We can lose with a hand of "good" cards; but even when dealt "bad" cards, one may be able to win. The process may have gone wrong from a genetic or technological perspective, but that does not mean it was a failure in a wider sense. When problems loom, so do opportunities. When things go "wrong" in someone's life, career, or marriage, that does not mean this person is a "lost cause" who does not deserve to live. Who has the right to claim that there are some human lives unworthy of living? Each setback may open the prospect of a comeback. As William Jennings Bryan used to say, "Destiny is not a matter of chance; it is a matter of choice."

Unfortunately, there is a biological notion called "survival of the fittest" which has brainwashed many biologists and physicians into assessing everything in terms of "winners" and "losers"—only the "fittest" are supposed to survive, and the others are considered "misfits." Surely, people with disabilities would, or should, vehemently protest upon hearing such statements. But are people with Down syndrome or any other chromosomal "disorder" really "losers"? They only would be if we place the final end of human beings solely in their biological worth. Yet, even those who vehemently herald diversity in society—which is considered "politically correct"—have no compunction about promoting the policy of uniformity of the "fittest." But is there not much more to life than biological worth? Just ask people with mental or physical disabilities whether they feel worthless. If they do say yes, it is most likely other people who have made them feel that way. When a blind woman was asked how she could be so joyful with her blindness, she responded with the question, "How can you see and *not* be joyful?"

Nevertheless, many scientists would tell you that chromosomal aberrations and other kinds of changes in genetic material are "random," and are therefore a matter of pure luck—in their view, bad luck. Later on in this book, we will discuss how random "randomness" really is (in Chapter 2). For now, it suffices to say that some scientists talk about randomness as if it were a deity with a capital R—but that is more of a world-view notion, certainly not a scientific concept. What they have in mind is the goddess of fate or doom. But there is no space for deities in science—or at least there should not be. Those who still maintain there is fate and doom in science are no longer teaching science but preaching science, making themselves the prophets of cynicism or nihilism. Those who confuse "random" with terms such as "ill-fated" or "unlucky" may be scientists but they are not speaking scientifically.

Apart from a scientific perspective, there are many other perspectives on human life. One of them is that humans live in a world of "good" and "evil." When we speak of evil, we are asserting somehow that evil should not exist. We are in fact evaluating physical suffering as wrong or bad—something no animal would be able to do. Prey does not consider the predator "evil"—perhaps painful, literally, but not evil. When giving birth, animals may experience physical pain, but not suffering in the sense of something "bad" or "evil." Only humans take genetic and other diseases as something that should not be, as something that seems to be acting against them personally. Animals may "dislike" these things, but they do not question them in terms of "Why *me*?" They do not have a "me," and since animals do not know about good and bad, they cannot ask why bad things happen to good animals. Humans, on the other hand, know what the world "should" be like, but only if they look at it from a "God's-eye" point of view. We know of "evil" because we have an idea of "good" and of what things should be like if everything were good—the way God had intended them to be.

It is also the "religious eye" that discerns God's gift in any newborn baby, regardless of its genetic makeup. As Pope Emeritus Benedict XVI put it in his first homily as Pontiff, "We are not some casual and meaningless product of evolution. Each of us is the result of a thought of God." To think differently will eventually lead to what C.S. Lewis called "the abolition of man." As Pope John Paul II once observed, "When the sense of God is lost, there is also a tendency to lose the sense of man, of his dignity and life." Human life starts "at the beginning" thanks to God's creation "in the beginning."

2

Life in the Womb

THE BIOLOGY BEHIND IT

In human beings, the egg cell is fertilized soon after ovulation, while it is still in the upper portion of the oviduct. Once the egg cell has been fertilized by a sperm cell, the development of a new organism begins. This is a process of staggering complexity, of which we only understand tiny parts. Humans possess a total of approximately 10^{14} (100 trillion) cells, consisting of more than 200 differentiated cell types. Starting from a single cell—the fertilized egg cell—all these diverse cell types have to be produced and organized into tissues and organs. The fertilized egg cell starts this process with the rapid proliferation of new cells through cell division or cleavage—exponentially, from one to two, from two to four, from four to eight, from eight to sixteen, and so forth, up to 100 trillion. In a sense, each one of us is a "self-made man."

From One Cell to Trillions of Cells

The sperm cell is an unusually small cell containing primarily DNA, with very little cytoplasm; most of the initial cytoplasm for the embryo comes from the relatively large egg cell, including its mitochondria, which are the "batteries" of the cell (carrying also their own mitochondrial DNA).

The penetration of a sperm cell into the egg cell stimulates the egg to begin development into an embryo. The penetration is the trigger event that induces the fusion of the sperm nucleus (including its DNA) with the egg nucleus (including its DNA). From then on, there is a new organism with a complete set of 23 pairs of chromosomes. Next, on the way to getting implanted in the uterine wall, the organism immediately begins cell cleavage.

Theoretically, we know that fertilization is the beginning of a new life; but the mother may not exactly know when the new life in her womb actually started. So how are days, weeks, and months counted from now on? When physicians talk about pregnancy, they often use two different terms—gestational age and fetal age. Gestational age refers to the length of time since the first day of a woman's last period. So, when the doctor says the gestational age is four weeks, it just means that it has been four weeks since the last menstrual period started.

Fetal age, on the other hand, refers to the "real" age of the developing baby, counting from the estimated date of conception. Since ovulation usually takes place two weeks after menstruation, the fetal age is typically two weeks less than the gestational age. So when using the gestational method of dating a pregnancy, one would technically be two weeks pregnant before conception even occurred. A full-term pregnancy lasts about 38 weeks, but since the expected delivery date is calculated from the first day of the last period, the entire pregnancy is said to have lasted 40 weeks, not 38. In what follows, ages given are "real" ages—fetal ages, that is (so two more weeks must be added to get gestational ages).

Once the growing fertilized egg cell has been imbedded into the uterine lining, the developing baby—often referred to as the embryo—goes through intense basic growth, beginning the development of the brain, spinal cord, heart, and gastrointestinal tract. During weeks two and three, arm and leg buds are visible, although not clearly distinguishable. The embryo lies inside the amniotic sac, bathed with amniotic fluid. By the twenty-third day, the outer embryonic membrane (the chorion) has merged with maternal tissues of the uterus to create a functional placenta, which produces the hormone hCG (human chorionic gonadotropin) to keep the production of progesterone going for the lining of the uterus; hCG can now be detected in urine and blood pregnancy tests.

By this time, the neural groove at the dorsal side of the embryo is complete and the tubular embryonic heart has begun to pulsate weakly, so there is movement of rudimentary blood through the main vessels. The early structures that will become the eyes and ears are forming. The embryo is a quarter-inch long by the end of the fourth week. The mother may not even know that she is pregnant yet, although it has been six weeks since her last period.

By the end of the first month, there are arm and leg buds, even hands and feet, but they are still mitten-like, with no separations between the individual fingers and toes. The neural tube at the dorsal side should be closed by now. During the fifth week, every essential organ has begun to form in the embryo's tiny body. During the sixth week, the ears are continuing to form externally and internally. In the eight week, all organs are functioning. Everything present in a human adult is now present in this tiny human being. The bones are beginning to form, and the muscles can contract. The facial features continue to mature, and the eyelids are now more developed. The embryo is about one inch long and is only the size of a bean.

From the ninth week on, medical professionals speak no longer of an embryo but of a fetus. At this time, the unborn child—as I prefer to call him or her—has grown to about three inches in length, and weighs about one ounce. We begin to see a human face with widely separated eyes and well-distinguished fingers and toes. The fingers now have permanent, individually unique fingerprints. Pain sensors begin to develop in the face of the unborn child. The genitalia have clearly formed into male or female, but still cannot be seen clearly on an ultrasound. The eyelids close and will not reopen until the twenty-sixth week after conception. The fetus can make a fist, and the buds for baby teeth appear. The head is nearly half the size of the entire new human being. The cerebral cortex has begun a crucial process of development.

During this time, outside factors can cause serious aberrations. Well-known are the disastrous effects of the infamous tranquilizer thalidomide when taken by the mother early in pregnancy. But in addition, generally mild viral diseases such as measles (rubella) can result in a malformed heart, deafness, or cataracts of the baby's eyes. Other potentially harmful infections include the cytomegalovirus (CMV), toxoplasmosis, and several sexually transmitted diseases such as syphilis, gonorrhea, and genital herpes. During this critical time, even a lack of the B-vitamin folic acid (folate) may cause the neural tube to not fully close, which leads to spina bifida.

By the end of 14 weeks, spontaneous muscle movements have become more frequent and can be felt by the mother more often. The cerebral hemispheres have begun to overlap the rest of the brain, and the sense organs are almost completely developed. Gradually the eyes will become light-sensitive and the ears audio-sensitive. During this time, many new brain cells are produced and new neural circuits established.

From week 15 through 18, the eyebrows and eyelashes grow in, and tiny nails begin to grow on the fingers and toes. The skin of the new human being is going through many changes and starts to produce a white pasty substance that covers the baby's skin to protect it from amniotic fluid. A fetal heartbeat can now be heard by a stethoscope. Sensory receptors develop all over the child's body. When provoked by painful stimuli, such as a needle, the unborn baby reacts, as can be measured by increases in the child's stress hormones, heart rate, and blood pressure. The unborn child has now reached a length of 8 inches and weighs about 12 ounces.

From weeks 19 through 21, the unborn baby is beginning to take on the look of a newborn infant as the skin becomes less transparent and fat begins to develop. All the components of the eyes are developed. The liver and pancreas are working hard to develop completely. The unborn baby has reached about 10–11 inches in length and weighs about 1–1¼ pounds.

From weeks 22 through 24, the baby could survive with the assistance of medical technology if it were delivered now. It has developed sleeping and waking cycles, and the mother will begin to notice when each of these takes place. The brain will be developing rapidly over the next few weeks. The nervous system has developed enough to control basic functions. The baby has reached about 14 inches in length and weighs about 2¼ pounds.

During weeks 25 through 30, the unborn baby really fills out, storing fat on the body, reaching about 15–17 inches in length, and weighing about 4–4½ pounds at the end of this period. The lungs are not fully mature yet, but some rhythmic breathing movements are occurring. Although the bones are fully developed, they are still soft and pliable. The eyelids open now—after having been closed since the end of the first trimester.

Beginning in week 31, the unborn baby descends into the head-down position in preparation for birth. It is beginning to gain weight more rapidly and is now 16–19 inches, weighing anywhere from 5¾ to 6¾ pounds. At 38 weeks of age, the baby is considered full-term and will be ready to make its appearance at any time. Its mother may notice fewer movements as the baby is now filling the uterus, with little room left to move. At this time, the mother is supplying her unborn baby with antibodies that will help protect against certain diseases. All organs are developed, with the lungs maturing all the way until the day of delivery. The baby is about 19–21 inches in length and weighs anywhere from 6¾ to 10 pounds.

Once it is time for birth, the birth process can be complicated by various factors. One of them is called placenta previa, in which the placenta has developed low in the uterus—either near, or sometimes above, the cervix. This condition occurs in about 1 out of 200 pregnancies. Sometimes, the placenta will still move up the wall of the uterus to a more normal position; if not, a caesarean section may be recommended.

Another potential problem is known as "mal-presentation." During delivery, the most frequent presenting part is the head, with the face towards the mother's back; this makes for the easiest passage through the birth canal. However, if the face is towards the mother's front, the baby cannot flex the neck to get around the curve of the birth canal; delivery by forceps might be required. Another complication can arise when the baby comes down the birth canal buttocks-first, so one or both feet may appear first. Such a delivery may require a Caesarian section as well. There is at least one more possible complication: the mother's pelvic cavity may be too narrow for the passage of her baby's head, or the baby's head abnormally large, as in hydrocephalus. Usually a Caesarian section is the best solution in such cases.

Even when there are no complications at the time of delivery, various dramatic changes must take place for every baby at the moment of birth. The placental circulation must be cut off; the temporary connection between the pulmonary artery and the aorta needs to be closed; any temporary openings in the wall between the left and right heart ventricle and between the left and right atrium are closed; the lungs are inflated for the first time; and blood is forced into the pulmonary circulation system. We all have gone through this process successfully, and hopefully unharmed. But let us not forget that, for nine months, we were confined to our mother's womb; it was in that small and intimate world that we shared her voice, her hormones, her food, her moods, perhaps even her nicotine, her alcohol, and her medications. There is growing evidence that when a pregnant woman goes through anger or depression during pregnancy, this experience has a lasting emotional and psychological effect on the child.

Most of the above processes—except for their time-frames—are not unique for us humans. We find them more or less with other mammals, and even to a certain degree with other vertebrates. The resemblances to other animals are most striking in the early embryonic stages, but they diminish in later stages when more distinctive human traits become apparent. This observation has made some people think that, during the embryological process, we repeat the process of evolution—from simple to more complex organisms. Indeed, we often do find intermediary stages of embryological development that were once final stages in more primitive animals. Human embryos, for instance, develop gill pouches just like fish, although they never become real gills; and the human cerebrum develops last. Also, human embryos still grow a layer of downy hair that they shed after about thirty-five weeks of gestation.

However, all this does not mean that human embryos are retracing the whole evolutionary history of humanity as they develop. The human embryo never has real gills in any sense of the word. The fanciful notion of such human gills is based upon the presence of six alternating ridges and grooves in the neck-region of the human embryo. While similar arches do give rise to gills in certain aquatic vertebrates such as fish, their development in mammals has nothing to do with gills or even breathing. In humans and other mammals, these arches and pouches develop into part of the face and its jaws (the first arch; a faulty closing of this arch would cause a cleft palate), muscles of facial expression (the second arch), some endocrine glands (the third and fourth arches), and the larynx (the sixth arch), whereas the fifth arch in fact disappears.

How long it takes for a new organism to grow in the womb is an altogether different issue. In the animal world we find that some mammals—typically herd animals—have a long growing process in the womb, so that they come out rather well developed; they can run around, follow the herd, and feed themselves as soon as they are born. Other mammals—typically nest animals—are born while still at an early stage of development, which makes them totally dependent on parental care in the nest.

Human beings fit in best with the latter group of organisms. We have to go through a long process of post-natal development, up to at least twenty years, and need lots of parental care in the "nest" at home. In the next two sections, we will discuss what this entails. But the great length of our post-natal process does not take away from the fact that our time in the womb has an enormous impact on the person we end up being. The pre-natal period seems to be a major factor that shapes the rest of our lives.

The Nervous System

An incredibly essential part of the development in the womb concerns the growth of the central nervous system—which is composed of the brain and the spinal cord. This system basically matures in a sequence from "tail" to head. In the fifth week after conception, the first neural connections begin forming in the spinal cord. By the sixth week, these early neural connections permit the first fetal movements which can be detected through ultrasound imaging.

Many other movements soon follow—of the limbs (around eight weeks) and fingers (ten weeks), as well as some surprisingly coordinated actions (hiccupping, stretching, yawning, sucking, swallowing, grasping, and thumb-sucking). By the end of the first trimester, the unborn baby has a remarkably rich repertoire of movements, even though most pregnant women still cannot feel any of them. They usually do not sense any movements of their unborn baby until the latter is 16 weeks old.

The second trimester marks the onset of other critical reflexes: continuous breathing movements (that is, rhythmic contractions of the diaphragm and chest muscles) and coordinated sucking and swallowing reflexes. These abilities are controlled by the brainstem, which sits above the spinal cord but below the higher, more complex cerebral cortex. The brainstem is responsible for many of our body's most vital functions, such as heart rate, breathing, and blood pressure. It is largely mature by the end of the second trimester, which is when babies first become able to survive outside the womb.

Last of all to mature is the cerebral cortex, which is responsible for most of what we think of as "mental life"—conscious experience, voluntary actions, thinking, remembering, and feeling. It has only begun to function around the time gestation comes to an end. Premature babies show only very basic electrical activity in the primary sensory regions of the cerebral cortex—in those areas that perceive touch, vision, and hearing—as well as in primary motor regions of the cerebral cortex. It develops progressively after birth.

In the last trimester, an unborn baby is capable of simple forms of learning, like habituation to a repeated auditory stimulus, such as a loud clap just outside the mother's abdomen. Shortly before birth, babies also seem to learn about the sensory qualities of the womb, since several studies have shown that newborn babies respond to familiar odors (such as their own amniotic fluid) and sounds (such as a maternal heartbeat or their own mother's voice). In spite of these rather sophisticated abilities, babies enter the world with a still rather primitive cerebral cortex, and it is the gradual maturation of this complex part of the brain that explains much of their emotional and cognitive maturation in the first few years of life (see the next section).

With the development of the nervous system, the senses develop in tandem. Not surprisingly, touch is the first sense to emerge in the dark environment of the womb; the baby wants to feel around and get the lay of the land. High-tech scanning has revealed that babies use touch to explore their body before birth. In the first trimester they can recognize sensations on the lips and nose. Tasting is next. By the second trimester, babies start to taste the amniotic fluid that surrounds them—and what the mother eats affects the flavor of the amniotic fluid and breast milk. By about 18 weeks, babies can hear; around 36 weeks, they are actively listening. What they are picking up is not only the background noise of the mother's heart, stomach, and intestines, but also what the mother says. The last development is the sense of vision. A baby's eyes are closed until about the 26th week of pregnancy, but when the eyelids are opened in this dark environment, enough light seeps in during the final two months for the baby to see its own leg and hand movements. Eventually, the baby will be ready to leave this quiet, warm, and dark womb for a loud, bright, open world—certainly a shocking contrast.

Sex Determination

What determines whether the new organism will be a female or a male? Rather complex mechanisms are responsible for sex determination and differentiation. In males, for instance, the steps of formation of the testes are dependent on a series of Y-linked and X-linked (among others) gene actions and interactions. Typically, sexual development is the result of numerous genes, whereas mutations in any of these genes can result in partial or complete failure of sex differentiation.

A simplified explanation would run as follows. As discussed earlier, the egg cell always carries one X-chromosome, but the sperm cell can introduce either an X- or a Y-chromosome. If fertilization is by a Y-bearing sperm cell, the new organism will usually develop into a male (XY). Hence, a baby's sex is determined at the time of conception. It is "genetic" in a rather odd sense. Whereas tall parents may have tall children, and short parents may have short children, every girl and every boy have exactly one parent of each sex. Because X-bearing and Y-bearing sperm cells should be equally common, we expect a 1:1 sex ratio. However, there are slight deviations from this expectation at birth. In almost all human populations of newborns, there is a slight excess of males—about 106 boys are born for every 100 girls. Part of the explanation might be a small difference in the ability of X-bearing and Y-bearing to fertilize egg cells and some difference in prenatal mortality rates between male and female fetuses.

Apparently the human Y-chromosome carries genes with strong male-determining properties; it is its absence that determines femaleness. However, it is not just the Y-chromosome itself that is the determining factor, but rather the *SRY* gene on the Y-chromosome which acts like a master switch and is responsible for the development of an unborn baby into a male by initiating the testes' development (whereas other genes on the Y-chromosome are important for male fertility). When this *SRY* gene is present, early embryonic testes do develop around the tenth week of pregnancy. In the absence of both the *SRY* gene and a testis-determining factor (*TDF*), ovaries develop. In general, one can say that sex determination depends on the testes, and testis-differentiation depends on the Y chromosome.

In the early developmental stages, the genitalia of males and females are virtually identical. Whether these structures will become female or male depends on the presence of the male hormone testosterone during this critical stage of development—more precisely, di-hydro-testosterone (DHT), a derivative of testosterone. In the absence of male hormone, the unborn baby develops as a female, no matter whether the Y-chromosome is present or not. At 10 weeks, the penis of the male is slightly larger than the clitoris of the female. At 12 weeks, the male scrotum has formed from the tissue that becomes the labia major in the female. Finally, at 34 weeks, the distinctive features of the genitalia of the two sexes are fully apparent. The anatomical differences between male and female are unambiguous at birth. Further differentiations take place during puberty (see Chapter 3).

The process described here is the normal means of sex differentiation. However, there can also be exceptional hormonal circumstances that change the way that the sex organs develop in males and females. For instance, some males have tissues that lack sensitivity to androgens, meaning they do not respond normally to the hormones that cause masculinization. Another example is when some females have overactive adrenal glands. This produces extra cortisol, a hormone that is structurally and functionally similar to testosterone. This is caused by recessive alleles that can also be found in males; they do not have a large impact. Then there are males with 5-? reductase deficiency. The enzyme 5-? reductase helps to control proportions of male sex hormones in the body. When there is not enough of this enzyme, normal sex differentiation does not occur.

Aside from these rare cases, it is the mere presence or absence of a Y-chromosome—or, more precisely, its *SRY* gene—that acts as a switch, early in development, to shunt the unborn baby into either one of two alternative developmental tracks, male or female. The rest is history.

BEHIND THE BIOLOGICAL FACTS

The complexity and precision characterizing the developmental changes we described in the previous section are staggering to contemplate. To mention just one example, approximately 43 muscles, 29 bones, and hundreds of nervous pathways must form in each human arm and hand alone. To function properly, all these components must be precisely correlated and coordinated. Incredibly sensitive mechanisms of developmental control must be at work for such an intricate structure to arise from a mass of initially undifferentiated cells. It is even much more amazing that all of this usually goes right than that it may sometimes go "wrong."

Why do things usually go *right* during the human development in the womb? A common answer to this question is that it took evolution millions of years to get it right. Why do most people accept such an answer? Because evolution is believed to work on a basis of natural selection—a process that selects and favors those mutated alleles that give the best results. Since mutations are presumable random, the whole process is considered random, fortuitous, and coincidental. How true is this conclusion?

How Random Is Random?

What do scientists mean when they call mutations "random"? The word "random" has many connotations. Usually we can replace the phrase "at random" with the expression "by chance," because they are basically interchangeable terms. So, in what sense do things in biology happen "by chance"?

It is common parlance in biology to state that mutations in genetic material happen "by chance." What scientists mean by this is, first of all, that mutations are unpredictable—as far as we know—in when and where they strike. We may know more nowadays about what exactly causes mutations (factors such as radiation, chemicals, free radicals, etc.), but we still cannot predict at what location in the DNA molecule those factors will hit and what changes they might generate there. They may not be unpredictable in principle, but they surely are in practice.

What else could scientists mean when talking about random mutations? They also mean that mutations are "unrelated," since there is no connection with anything else that is going on (other than radiation or chemical pollutants). In addition, they mean that mutations are somehow "arbitrary," because they do not select their target but hit indiscriminately—"good" and "bad" spots alike. Finally, they mean that mutations are just "opportunistic," because they occur without reference to any particular outcome, let alone because of any specific future needs. There is no physical mechanism that detects which mutations would be beneficial and then causes those mutations to occur. But that is where randomness ends.

Natural selection, on the other hand, is far from being random in the way mutations are. Natural selection only happens "by chance" in one particular sense: it makes a group of organisms adapt to a volatile environment, without regard for the changes the future will bring. When the environment changes, certain adaptations may no longer be appropriate; so in retrospect we may consider these adaptations rather "opportunistic" and short-sighted. Yet, natural selection, in and of itself, is highly selective, and definitely not random in the sense of arbitrary.

Apparently, the process of natural selection—though based on (random) mutations—is, even when taken in its entirety, not really random in the strict sense, because natural selection can only select those biological designs that are in accordance with what may be called the *cosmic design*. Eyes, hearts, and brains "work" because they follow the chemical and physical laws laid down in the cosmic design of this universe. The universe has an overall set of restraints harnessing individual designs and making them "fit" and "successful" to a certain degree—in contrast to designs that are less "successful."

Without a cosmic design in the "background," the biological

design of a heart could not work at all. So it is no wonder that the working of a heart has to follow hydrodynamic and electromagnetic laws. The wing of a bird, as another example, follows the same laws of aerodynamics as the wing of a plane—and fish follow the same hydrodynamic laws as submarines. Whatever follows the correct laws—which are part of the cosmic design—will likely succeed. In the words of physician and scientist Leon Kass, there is "something" in successful biological designs that carries them through the filter of natural selection. In other words, natural selection on its own cannot do its "job" unless it works within a framework of cosmic design. Natural selection can only select those specific *biological* designs that follow the rules of the *cosmic* design (just as designers, engineers, and architects must do). That does not sound very random to me. Put differently, Darwinism could never survive without the concept of design—whether Darwinists realize this or not.

Ultimately, there may not be as much "chance" in evolution as some would suggest. And let me add one more cautious note: some people would like to take the notion of randomness to an entirely different level, the level of a worldview. They take chance or randomness to be another name for some kind of capricious, blind agent called fate. It would be more appropriate to label this as "chance with a capital C" or "randomness with a capital R"—the goddess of Fate, or Blind Fate, or Doom.

Those who take the word *chance* out of its scientific context and interpret it as meaning "senseless," "meaningless," or "blind" are actually changing "lower-case chance" into "upper-case Chance"—a capricious, blind agent, actually a deity, or a "blind watchmaker" at best, that turns the whole of life into a mere play of whimsical and fortuitous events. But there is no room for deities in science. Those who speak in such terms may be scientists, but they are certainly not speaking scientifically. The notion of "luck" does not belong to a scientist's vocabulary—it is a philosophical notion, associated with concepts such as doom, fate, and misfortune—and in stark contrast to concepts such as destiny, blessing, and divine intervention.

Those who speak of "bad luck" consider the thing or event in question as a failure, as something that they dislike, condemn, or even reject—in short, as something that *should* not be. However,

41

judgments about what should be and should not be go far beyond science and beyond a scientist's competence—they are actually *moral* evaluations and judgments, often with a religious or semi-religious undertone (see Chapter 4). What some call a curse may actually turn out to be a blessing, for each setback may open up the prospect of a comeback.

Even if one believes that we are products of evolution, such a belief in itself does not imply that we are products of blind fate. And most religious believers would add to this that nothing is really random in this world anyway, when seen from a religious, divine perspective. As the physicist Stephen Barr noted, when we speak of randomness in science, we are speaking of how things in this universe are related to each other—not how they are related to God. When it comes to God, randomness loses its meaning. As St. Padre Pio would say, it is God who arranges the coincidences. Once he asked a man who claimed that a certain event had happened by chance: "And who, do you suppose, arranged the chances?" Science has no answer to this question—not even the answer "nobody did." Anything that seems to be random from a scientific point of view may very well be included in God's eternal plan. As a matter of fact, St. Thomas Aquinas once said, "Whoever believes that everything is a matter of chance, does not believe that God exists."

Returning to the issue of conception and pre-natal development, the DNA behind these processes is not a product of blind fate either. It has gone through a long evolutionary process in which it has been fine-tuned and perfected in accordance with the laws of the cosmic design. As I stated earlier, the complexity and precision of all these developmental changes are staggering to contemplate. Incredibly sensitive mechanisms of developmental control must operate together for such an intricate structure as that of a human being to arise from a "simple" egg cell with its DNA and a "simple" sperm cell with its DNA. There is not much "randomness" left now. Not much in life is left to mere chance—let alone to blind destiny.

A Human Being in the Making
Each human being is genetically the same individual at every stage of life's journey, in spite of changes in appearance—a *human* being

from the very beginning; not complete yet, but definitely in the making. At the moment of conception, the new being could say, "I am a boy," or "I am a girl"—and that's how it will stay. From fertilization on, life's journey is a continuum, so there is no such thing as a "pre-embryonic phase," let alone a "pre-human stage," in this process. Even when we use terms such as "embryo," "fetus," or "unborn baby," in all such instances we are referring to steps in one long, continuous developmental growth process that starts with a fertilized egg cell outfitted with human chromosomes and human DNA. What remains the same during the entire process of adding, replacing, and losing cells is the person's identity, the person's soul. Humans have the capacity to change without losing their identity. Although our bodies change constantly, we ourselves do not—that is, our personal identity remains the same. In a certain sense, the body is not only something we *have*, but also something we *are*.

If this is true, then a human being does not just start begin to *become* human at a specific stage in its growing process, but rather *is* already human from the very beginning. Human life is a journey that does not start halfway. An unborn baby cannot be "half human" any more than a woman can be "half pregnant." From this follows an important conclusion. A new human being does not *become* human at some point during its development, but rather *is* uniquely human at every stage of its growth process—which is partially due to the fact that its DNA is human from the very beginning. As Pope Francis put it in his apostolic exhortation *Evangelii Gaudium*, "a human being is always sacred and inviolable, in any situation and at every stage of development. Human beings are ends in themselves and never a means of resolving other problems." We are a unique human being from the very day of our conception.

When calling an organism "human," we can have two very different things in mind. On the one hand, the word *human* can be a descriptive qualification in terms of biology; an organism is called human because it came from human beings, its DNA is human, its developmental path is human, its anatomy and physiology are human, and it belongs to the human race. This sense of the word is descriptive in the same way as the word *normal* can describe what the norm, the average, or the standard is.

On the other hand, the word *human* also has a moral or ethical connotation. In that specific sense, it is not of a descriptive but of a prescriptive nature. Calling a being "human," in this prescriptive sense, means that it has human qualifications, including human rights, and therefore deserves human protection and merits to be treated as human—and, hence, to think differently would be "inhuman." This sense of the word is prescriptive in the same way as the world *normal* can also prescribe what is considered normal as opposed to abnormal. This is a matter of morality. Moral prescriptions are not descriptions, but they tell us what we owe others—our duties—and what others owe us—our rights (see Chapter 4).

However, the problem with moral prescriptions is that they do not coincide with biological descriptions. We cannot define moral notions in non-moral terms; propositions containing terms that apply to morality cannot be deduced from propositions in which moral terms are missing. The fact that something *is* a certain way does not entail that it *ought* to be that way; the fact that diseases are "natural" in a biological sense does not entail they are "good" in a moral sense; the fact that there is biological development does not mean there is also a development in human dignity. The fact that some people are richer than others, or more intelligent than others, does not mean that we ought to value them differently in a moral sense. They may have more power than others, but they should not have more rights than others.

Nevertheless, the putative value of human life has often been based on the use of biological criteria, such as the extent of cerebral activity. For some, this kind of quasi-moral argument would go along the following lines: The more cerebral activity there is, the more value a human being has, and therefore, the more rights it has and the more protection it deserves. For others, the criterion that determines the humanity of an unborn child is viability—the more viable, the more human. However, the biological criteria adduced here are biological descriptions and do not ipso facto qualify as moral prescriptions.

The development in the womb is a continuum, as we have seen. Embryos do not spontaneously transform into human beings at the moment their senses start to function, any more than they spontaneously transform into human beings at the moment their hearts start to beat, or their limbs start to move, or their brains begin to function—each of which occurs at different points along the child's normal path of growth and development. To use an analogy, the monarch butterfly goes through dramatic changes from egg to caterpillar, to pupa, and finally to a mature butterfly, but it remains a member of the species *Danaus plexippus* all the way through. One and the same entity may go through various *appearances*, but it remains the same entity.

Some people think of human rights as if they were entitlements that the government gives us. Indeed, we gain entitlements as we age—we can drive a car at sixteen, we can vote at eighteen, we can drink alcohol at twenty-one. But we cannot apply this kind of reasoning to human rights. A human being does not gain more rights when it progresses further along the path toward being born. Protection of a human being is not a conditional legal entitlement, but an unconditional moral right. It does not increase with age, but is rooted in the fact that we are dealing with a human being from the very beginning. There is no gradualism when it comes to human rights; killing a twenty-year-old is not worse than killing a fourteen-year-old. Moral status and human development are not linked that way. There is a fundamental difference between the moral right to life and the legal entitlements we are given to vote or drive.

The neuroscientist and bioethicist Fr. Tadeusz Pacholczyk uses the thalidomide drama of the late 1950s and early 1960s to clarify that if it were true that women are not pregnant with a human being prior to the eighth week of gestation, then taking a drug like thalidomide would not raise any concerns, since no human being would be present to be harmed by the drug anyway. But it is well known that the most drug-susceptible period of pregnancy is the first trimester, specifically between the fourth and the seventh weeks of gestation. Apparently, each human being begins at fertilization and consists as a biological continuum thereafter. Upon fusion with a sperm cell, the egg cell as egg no longer exists, and a human being—genetically distinct from his or her mother—starts a new life's journey. I know, for instance, that I myself started at one point in my life as a fertilized egg cell, and that at some point in time I will be dead. It is my very "self" that connects all the stages of my life in one long continuum.

In other words, the moral quality of human life is not a biological issue. It cannot be quantified and measured on a scale; it does not depend on the degree of cerebral activity, for example. We cannot use relative standards of intelligence, viability, maturity, health, fitness, and the like to measure or judge the absolute moral value of human life. Biological standards are of a quantitative nature, and thus can be put on a scale; but moral standards are of a qualitative nature and cannot be rated or ranked.

Put differently, we cannot use biological criteria to make a moral decision—something like "the adult is more important than the unborn baby," or "an independent human life outweighs a dependent human life," or "a full-grown person is worth more than a growing fetus," "a full-grown brain is worth more than a brain in development," "a life in the womb has fewer rights than a life in the cradle," "a perfect embryo is worth more than an imperfect embryo"—the list could go on and on. Human status and human dignity are not something to be earned—they are given. Being of human descent is enough; you can neither earn nor forfeit your humanity. If the death of a baby, either born or unborn, does not matter, then no human death matters.

Let me explain this point further with an example used by Abraham Lincoln in discussing the issue of slavery. In his own, rather technical words,

> If A. can prove, however conclusively, that he may, of right, enslave B.—why may not B. snatch the same argument, and prove equally, that he may enslave A?—You say A. is white, and B. is black. It is color, then; the lighter, having the right to enslave the darker? Take care. By this rule, you are to be slave to the first man you meet, with a fairer skin than your own. You mean the whites are intellectually the superiors of the blacks; and, therefore have the right to enslave them? Take care again. By this rule, you are to be slave to the first man you meet, with an intellect superior to your own.

Lincoln's point is clear: All the answers you might come up with to defend your moral claim use relative criteria—which are at any rate morally irrelevant—such as a darker skin color or a lower intelligence. Because those criteria are relative, they would entail that someone with a lighter skin or higher intelligence would have the "moral right" to enslave you. And the same holds for the moral value of human life. This value cannot be based on biological standards, since those are per definition morally irrelevant, and relative besides. In contrast, moral values are absolute ends-in-themselves—not disposable means-to-other-ends. Whereas our bodily movements are subject to physical constraints, our actions are subject to moral ones.

Once we realize that the word "human" does not only mean "belonging to the human race" but also "having human rights," we might take a different look at various forms of in-vitro-fertilization (IVF). Fr. Tadeusz Pacholczyk argued against the morality of IVF by claiming that our children have the *right* to be procreated, not produced. They have the *right* to come into the world in the personal, love-giving embrace of their parents, not in the cold and impersonal glass world of a test tube or Petri dish. They have the *right* to be uniquely, exclusively, and directly related to the mother and father who bring them into the world. In-vitro-fertilization ignores and even violates all these moral rights of the child; it gives the embryo an "out-of-body" experience, so to speak.

Rights are what we owe others and what others owe us; they come with the fact that we—even as unborn babies—are human beings in the full sense. Duties and rights go hand in hand, so they have a natural reciprocity: children have the right to be born in a womb, so parents have the duty to make that happen for their children. Some might object that parents also have the right to have children, even if infertility makes that impossible. However, no one has the *right* to have children, for no one has the *duty* to have children. The Congregation of the Doctrine of the Faith (CDF) put it well in its 1987 instruction *Donum Vitae*: "The child is not an object to which one has a right, nor can he be considered as an object of ownership: Rather, a child is a gift, 'the supreme gift' and the most gratuitous gift of marriage." This document made it clear that we must not have babies without sex, whereas Pope Paul VI's 1968 encyclical *Humanae Vitae*, had already explained why we must not have sex without babies. There are clear harms and evils in the separation of sex from procreation. There is surely more to the discussion, but the above point is often completely neglected.

Let me end this chapter with the following question: Would there be any sanctuary left if even the womb of a pregnant mother is no longer a safe hiding place for new life? Women have received the power to give life, not to take life. Perhaps you remember the billboard in Manhattan that read, "The most dangerous place for African-Americans is in the womb." They count for 60% of the city's abortions. Some may write this off this as a racist remark, but it is actually taking a strong stand in defense of our black fellow-citizens—of all those black babies that were not allowed to be born. It is just a matter of fact that the womb is the most dangerous place for African Americans in New York City.

Genetic Testing

Genetic testing is developing at rocket pace in our society. Very recently, scientists developed a "chemical fingerprint" that identified twenty-two molecules linked to metabolism that may indicate how a person will grow old. Such testing, it was observed, could lead to innovative treatments for age-related conditions. This may be good news, although tests like these will not be readily available anytime soon. On the other hand, who is to know on what day a person is going to die, and of which disease? The research behind these tests is always based on probabilities, not certainties, so no one should or could play "God" in predicting someone else's destiny. Besides, one should consider what the effect of such "knowledge" would be. It could change life dramatically and make for self-fulfilling prophecies.

In this context, it is worth focusing on another, more popular development: *prenatal* genetic testing. Since the 1980's, doctors have extracted samples of the embryo's outer membrane (chorionic villus sampling, or CVS) and of the fluid inside the inner membrane (amniocentesis) to diagnose genetic diseases such as Tay-Sachs syndrome and Down syndrome before the baby is born.

First, a word of medical caution: there is a small risk that an amniocentesis could cause injury to the baby or mother, infection, or preterm labor. Both tests invade the womb for samples of fetal genetic material, so they carry risks of infection and miscarriage. In fact, amniocentesis can even cause the birth defect of clubbed feet.

Second, a word of theoretical caution: even though some genetic diseases may appear to be predetermined and inescapable when the genetic indicators are present, this is not always the case. Even if geneticists know that everyone with the disease has that one particular allele, they do not know whether there are people walking around with that same allele who never developed the disease. The designation of an allele as "dominant" should always be done very cautiously.

Then, a word of philosophical caution: to reiterate, we should not forget that there is no such thing as a "perfect" genome. If we do not want less-than-perfect children, no child would make the cut. Every day, researchers around the world report new disease-associated mutations in medical journals. Such studies show that we are all walking genetic "junkyards." Recent research suggests that every individual carries, on average, 313 disease-causing mutations. However, not all mutations cause diseases; and besides, diseases may very well be just part of life.

Moreover, we do not really know whether one allele is "better" than another allele—since so much depends on what the surrounding genes are and do. Everybody has genetic flaws; it just depends on how they become manifest in someone's life. If you are looking for something wrong, you will certainly find it. The real issue is whether we actually need that genetic information, and if so, what we do with it.

Recently, several firms began offering non-invasive blood tests for Down syndrome and for other forms of trisomy disorders in which there are three instead of two of the same chromosome (see Chapter 1). Further non-invasive tests have been developed that promise to scan the whole genome of the fetus for more than 3,000 single-gene disorders. It is clear what the outcome of such tests is: it will almost certainly expand the "genetic grounds" for abortion. As a matter of fact, most children with Down syndrome diagnosed in utero never experience a birthday. Three different studies have estimated abortion rates after genetic testing at 87%, 95%, and 98%.

One of the reasons for these high numbers is that the prenatal diagnosis of Down syndrome is often accompanied by negative information, followed by the suggestion to terminate the pregnancy. Recently, a national law (2008) and three state laws—in Virginia (2007), Missouri (2011), and Massachusetts (2012)—mandate that women receive up-to-date and scientific information on paper from their health care providers, and that they recommend a referral to support groups or support services providers.

Unquestionably, there is a lot of misinformation on Down-syndrome children, referring to them with dehumanizing labels. Nonetheless, whereas they used to be raised in institutions they are now mostly brought home. As a result, many of them drive, work, marry, and even hold college degrees. Their life expectancy has quintupled, increasing from 12 years in 1912 to 60 years in 2012. People who know them say there is something joyful, magnetic, and exuberant about them—even something therapeutic.

Then there is another side to genetic testing. It is almost inevitable that test results may be incorrect—so-called false positives. Incorrect test results may not only bring about wrong decisions, but will also lead to costly court rulings, which in turn will force companies to be mindful of the potential cost associated with any disability that arises, if it could have been tested for prior to birth. Eventually this may lead to forced pre-natal testing and forced abortion of babies with disabilities. We might be entering here the doom-scenario of *eugenics*—as it was announced in Aldous Huxley's *Brave New World*. But who decides if a newly discovered mutation goes on the eugenicists' list of unwanted diseases?

What does eugenics stand for? Eugenics basically asserts that we should breed humans like we breed animals—and that we may kill them like we kill animals. At the beginning of the previous century, eugenics flourished—not only at universities and on the editorial boards of scientific journals, but also in politics. Supreme Court Justice Oliver Wendell Holmes declared in Buck v. Bell (1927) that "three generations of imbeciles are enough," and launched a massive campaign of forced sterilizations. Eugenicists started giving IQ tests to Jewish immigrants on Ellis Island and reported that 40% of them were "feeble-minded." The 1924 Immigration Act drew heavily on ideas from eugenicists such as Madison Grant and Harry Laughlin. Eugenicists are cut from the same cloth as KKK members, as both groups reject human equality; they consider some better than others, or at least claim some should be treated better than others.

Eugenics may have been dormant for a while, but it came alive again as the major ideology behind our so-called Reproductive Genetic Technologies (RGT), often connected with in-vitro-fertilization procedures (IVF). Here we have a new breed of eugenicists who urge parents to have the "best" children by using what they call a pre-implantation genetic diagnosis (PGD). In this procedure, a single cell is extracted from an IVF embryo and then tested to see which embryos make the genetic cut. The embryos that "fail" the test are discarded or donated to research. The ones that "pass" have a chance to be transferred into a womb. Let us not defend this with the slogan "Man's power over Nature," for that is ultimately what C. S. Lewis called "a power exercised by some men over other men with Nature as its instrument."

All the technologies mentioned in this chapter are in essence modern versions of eugenics and were introduced so as to eventually eradicate diseases in the human race, not only by genetic engineering, but also by destroying human life. Their defenders cleverly swap one moral value, the sanctity of life, with another moral value, the prevention of suffering. Since words are inherently pliable, they can easily be adapted to any ideology. No wonder, some of these ideologists have put a nice label on this kind of abortion by calling it "eugenic abortion." Some have even chosen to label abortion as a "cure" for the "disease" of pregnancy. Then again, others call abortion and abortive contraceptives a "health-care" issue; but none of this has anything to do with the health of the mother, let alone the health of the aborted unborn baby. Pope John Paul II has drawn attention to the two radically different meanings of the word "my." When I say, "This is my phone," I mean I *own* the phone. On the other hand, when I say, "This is my wife," it is clear I am not claiming I own her, but I am *part* of her. The same holds for an unborn baby. The new person in the womb is not some*thing* the mother owns, but some*one* she is part of and responsible for. Parents are not owners of their children, but rather guardians or stewards.

Fortunately, there are also modern technologies with a positive impact. The use of ultrasounds, for instance, allows us to actually "see" what is growing in the womb, making a pregnant mother more aware of what—or rather who—is growing in the hidden recesses of her womb. There are currently 29 states that demand ultrasounds prior to abortions. It was the ultrasound that led former abortionist Dr. Bernard Nathanson to become pro-life as far back in 1979, when the first generation of ultrasounds convinced this man, a self-described "Jewish atheist" who was one of America's leading abortionists and co-founder of what is now NARAL Pro-Choice America, that he was killing unborn children.

Perhaps, though, genetic testing can also be a positive, useful tool to prepare parents for their special-needs children. More likely, however, it will provide another reason for "artificial selection" against young human beings with "imperfect" DNA, and for ending their lives prematurely. At the same time, it is basically conveying the message to existing people with disabilities that their lives are not worth living, that they should not have been. Surely, those people won't be very pleased to hear that message.

Interestingly enough, the man who discovered the cause of Down syndrome, Dr. Jérôme Lejeune, dedicated his entire career to protecting children with the syndrome by all the means at his disposal. In a similar vein, former Surgeon General C. Everett Koop worked endlessly for children with congenital defects. In 1976, after spending an entire Saturday with his pediatric surgery team operating on three patients with severe congenital defects, Koop sat in the cafeteria and remarked that together they had given over two hundred years of life to three individuals who together barely weighed ten pounds.

3

Growing Up

THE BIOLOGY BEHIND IT

It is a moment parents never forget—the first time they hold their new baby in their arms. Who is this mysterious new person? Before long, they will know more, as this baby grows up in their midst. But as much as they are learning, the new baby is learning a thousand times more. And before they know it, the little one will be grown up.

What happens during the growing-up process of life's journey actually covers several periods—early childhood (1–4), middle childhood (5–8), pre-adolescence (9–13), adolescence (14–17)—and it ends when "legal adulthood" sets in at 18–21 years, depending on the law of the land. Another term for the periods of pre-adolescence and adolescence combined is "puberty." Although puberty is only part of this entire stage of life's journey, it is probably the most turbulent part.

Actually, every part of this stage is a turbulent process. Considering how amazingly uncoordinated babies are at birth, it is a wonder they learn to walk at all. Even blind babies learn to walk—and they are certainly not imitating anyone. Children are just motivated by an irrepressible desire to reach beyond themselves. And something similar holds for many other processes of development during this stage. Here are some further details.

Some Milestones

Much of the further course of life depends on how a child began its own life on earth outside the womb. Children who were malnourished between mid-gestation and two years of age do not adequately grow, either physically or mentally. Even after birth, they lag behind in body growth and brain development. This should not surprise us, since a lot needs to be done in the first years of post-natal life, especially as far as growth in size is concerned. It seems like the body has to make up for the time of spatial confinement in the womb. The baby, and soon the little toddler, goes through a dramatic growth-spurt, which gradually slows down and then levels off at the age of 20.

However, growth does not occur at the same rate and at the same time in all parts of the body. The differences between a newborn baby and an adult human being are differences not only in overall size but also in proportions. The head of a young child is far larger in relation to the rest of its body than that of an adult. And the child's legs are much shorter in relation to its trunk than those of the adult. If the child's body were simply to grow as large as an adult's body, while maintaining the same proportions, the result would be a very un-adult-like individual. The head of an adult is only ⅛ of the total body-length, whereas it was ½ of the total body-length at 2 months after fertilization.

Normal adult proportions develop because the various parts of the body either grow at quite different rates or stop growing at different times. The same holds for internal organs. The heart keeps growing at the rate at which the body grows, but the brain has already reached its full size at the age of five—which, however, does not mean it stops maturing. But even inside the brain, there is proportional growth. It was discovered that the cerebral cortex, which is the wrinkled area on the surface of the brain responsible for higher mental functions, grows in an uneven fashion. Up to one-third of the cortex expands approximately twice as much as other cortical areas as an infant gradually matures into a young adult. The reason for this is not obvious. Perhaps the full physical growth of these regions may be somewhat delayed to allow them to be shaped by early life experiences. Another factor might be that, in order to pass through the mother's pelvis at birth, brain size had to be constrained, with its most important parts prioritized.

All the previous steps are necessary for the development of the child's physical and mental skills. These steps come in a certain order—for example, a child will not stand before having learned to sit. But the rate at which these skills are acquired varies enormously. Yet here are some rough averages for each milestone: smiling at 6 weeks; rolling over from a sideways position onto the back at 10 weeks; raising head and shoulders from a face-down position at 5 months; sitting up unsupported at 6 months; saying simple two-syllable words such as "Mama" and "Dada" at 8 months; trying to use a spoon at 8 months; rising to a sitting position at 9 months; understanding simple commands at 12 months; walking unaided at 18 months; achieving bowel control at 20 months; staying dry during the day at 2 years; talking in simple sentences at 3 years; getting dressed at 4 years.

These are all averages, so do not mark them on your calendar. When children develop these skills at a slower pace, there is usually no reason to panic. Everyone has heard of "late walkers" and "delayed talkers," but they will usually catch up—unless there is some underlying problem such as a hearing or vision problem. In order to learn to speak, a child must be able to hear others speaking. In order to learn to read, a child must be able to see clearly. We are not only what we eat, but also what we hear, see, and read.

This also means that parents should take an active role in speaking and reading to their infants and toddlers. The size of a toddler's vocabulary is strongly correlated with how much a mother talks to her child. But it has got to be "live" language, not television; language has to be used in a personal relationship—or it is just *noise*. Something similar holds for reading. Since only half of our toddlers are routinely read to by their parents, teachers have been reporting that more than a third of kindergartners are not ready to learn when they arrive at school. And unfortunately, some children do not speak because nobody speaks to them.

Brain Development

A significant part of this important stage in life is brain development. Although it has already undergone an amazing amount of development, the brain of a newborn baby is still very much a work-in-progress. It remains small—little more than one-quarter of its adult size. The sensory skills of babies at birth are just rudimentary. In the womb, they were already able to recognize their parents' voices, but their visual skills are still very limited just after birth; they can only focus on objects no farther than 13 inches away—about the distance to the mother's face when bottle- or breast-feeding. They can track slow-moving objects, but lose them when they are more than 18 inches away. For the first few weeks, this is all the vision they need—and about all that the brain can handle. How come?

By birth, only the lower portions of the nervous system (the spinal cord and brain-stem) are well-developed, whereas the higher regions (the limbic system and cerebral cortex) are still rather primitive. Because it takes time for the human brain to develop, nature has ensured that the neural circuits responsible for the most vital bodily functions—such as breathing, heartbeat, circulation, sleeping, sucking, and swallowing—are up and running by the time a baby emerges from the protective womb. The rest of the brain's development can follow at a more leisurely pace.

In spite of the great number of neurons present at birth, brain size itself increases rather gradually. A newborn's brain is only about one-fourth the size of an adult's, and then it grows to about 80% of adult size by age three and 90% by age five. This growth is largely due to changes in individual neurons, which are structured much like trees. Thus, each brain cell begins as a tiny sapling and only gradually sprouts its hundreds of long, branching dendrites. Brain growth is largely due to the growth of these dendrites, which serve as the receiving points for input from the long arms, called axons, of other neurons. This is the moment when connections between neurons are being made, which is called *synaptic* reorganization.

What does this reorganization entail? Synapses are the connecting points between the long axon of one neuron and the short dendrite of another. While information travels down the length of a single axon as an electrical signal, it has to be transmitted across the synapse through the release of tiny packets of chemicals, called neurotransmitters—from axon to dendrite. On the dendrite side, special receptors for neurotransmitters change the chemical signal into an electrical signal again, then repeating the process in the next neuron in the chain. The number of synapses in the cerebral cortex peaks within the first few years of life, but then declines by about one-third between early childhood and adolescence. This is known as *pruning*. Let me explain.

At its peak, the cerebral cortex creates an astonishing two-million new synapses every second. The brain actually over-produces connections—some 50% more than will be preserved in adulthood. With these new connections come a baby's many mental milestones, such as color vision and a pincer grasp (picking up objects with thumb and index finger). The number of synapses remains at this over-abundant level throughout middle childhood (4–8 years of age). But after that, the number of synapses gradually declines, reaching adult levels. However, this does not mean that the brain loses functionality; rather, it becomes more efficient due to the reduction of unused pathways.

So it is actually what a child experiences—in sensory, motor, emotional, and intellectual avenues—that determines which of these synapses will be preserved through pruning the least useful connections. In this way, each child's brain becomes better-tuned to meet the challenges of his or her particular environment. Pruning streamlines children's neural processing, so the remaining circuits work more quickly and efficiently. Since the adult human brain contains about 100 billion neurons linked by more than 100 trillion synapses, researchers are now developing ways to automate the mapping of this gigantic network of synapses—which is called the *Human Connectome Project*, comparable to the *Human Genome Project*.

A second important stage in the development of the brain is the period when axons, the long ends of neurons, are being insulated. A newborn's brain works at a considerably slower pace than an adult's, transmitting information some sixteen times less efficiently. But soon the speed of neural processing begins to improve dramatically during infancy and childhood, reaching its maximum around age 15. Most of this increase is due to the gradual *myelination* of the long axon "wires" that connect one neuron to another neuron's dendrites. Myelin is a very dense, fatty substance that insulates axons much like the plastic insulation on telephone wires, increasing the speed of electrical transmission and preventing cross-talk between adjacent nerve fibers—making sure that electrical signals do not leak out and dissipate.

This coating or covering of axons with myelin begins around birth and is most rapid during the first two years but continues perhaps as late as 30 years of age. Because of the rapid pace of myelination in early life, children need a high level of fat in their diets—for some, 50% of their total calories—including cholesterol, which makes up 20% of myelin. Not only does breast milk provide lots of cholesterol, it also provides a specific enzyme to allow the baby's digestive tract to absorb almost 100% of that cholesterol, necessary for a healthy development of brain and eyes—notwithstanding the anti-cholesterol rhetoric that we are presently being bombarded with.

Windows of Opportunity

While the brain goes through a process of growing and specializing, the young child goes through a process of learning. The brain is undeniably more "plastic" in early life than in maturity. This plasticity has both a positive and a negative side. On the positive side, it means that the brains of young children are more open to educational and enriching influences. Babies are learning machines; everything is interesting to them, so parents should take advantage of their child's natural curiosity. On the negative side, it also means that young children's brains are more vulnerable to developmental problems should their environment prove especially impoverished, under-nurturing, or traumatizing. As Bruce Perry, M.D., of Baylor College of Medicine, puts it: If the brain's organization reflects its experience, and the experience of the traumatized child is fear and stress, then the neurochemical responses to fear and stress become the most powerful architects of the brain. In short, brain development is an experience-dependent process.

If experiences are that important for brain development, the next question would be: What is the best time to learn? There seem to be certain periods when learning is crucial, or at least optimal. For instance, if babies do not receive normal visual input at an early age, they may suffer permanent impairment; in the same way, children born with crossed or "lazy" eyes will fail to develop full acuity and depth perception if the problem is not promptly corrected.

Something similar holds for language skills; they depend critically on verbal input in the first few years, in the absence of which certain skills, especially grammar and pronunciation, may be permanently impacted. This process does not just start in the nursery but has begun already in the womb, where the unborn baby was continually bathed in the sounds of its mother's voice. The critical period for language-learning begins to end around five years of age and is wholly finished by around puberty. This is the reason why individuals who learn a new language after puberty usually speak it, and keep speaking it, with a foreign accent.

In this context we should at least mention Jean Piaget (1896–1980), a biologist who originally studied mollusks but switched to the study of the development of children's understanding, through observing them with his biological acuity while talking and listening to them as they worked on exercises he designed. He came to distinguish four developmental stages. Nowadays his scheme is considered too rigid—many children manage concrete operations earlier than he had thought, and some people never attain formal operations, or at least are not called upon to use them—but his general idea is still valid: before they have reached a certain age, children are not capable of understanding things in certain ways. Here are those four stages:

1. Sensorimotor (birth–2 years): The child differentiates self from objects and recognizes the self as an agent of action who can act intentionally (e.g., pulling a string to set a mobile in motion or shaking a rattle to make a noise). The child realizes that things continue to exist even when they are no longer present to the senses.

2. Pre-operational (2–7 years): The child learns to use language and to represent objects by images and words. Thinking is still egocentric, so it is hard to take the viewpoint of others. The child is able to classify objects by a single feature (e.g., grouping together all red blocks regardless of shape, or all square blocks regardless of color).

3. Concrete operational (7–11 years): The child can think logically about objects and events, and achieves conservation of number (age 6), mass (age 7), and weight (age 9). Objects are classified

according to several features and can be ordered in a series by a single dimension, such as size.

4. Formal operational (11 years and up): Adolescents begin to think logically about abstract propositions and can test hypotheses systematically. They become concerned with hypothetical, upcoming, and ideological issues.

During these important formative years, things can go "wrong" in many ways: the educational environment may be impoverished, or the nutritional situation may be inadequate, or environmental factors may interfere; but there may also be biological defects. Sometimes it is hard to pinpoint the underlying factors. An important area of uncertainty is the so-called attention-deficit/hyperactivity disorder (ADHD), seemingly so rampant today. One particular neural structure of interest here has been the caudate nucleus, which is located in the center of the brain and is associated with the neurotransmitter dopamine. The caudate has been found to be smaller in children with ADHD, possibly indicating lower availability of dopamine—the neurotransmitter that assists with focusing of attention and impulse control. Other studies have also found smaller frontal lobe volumes in children with ADHD, in particular the white matter volume of the frontal lobe which is composed of nerve fibers. Differences have also been found in the white matter (composed of nerve fibers) in the posterior regions of the brain, particularly for those children who did not respond to stimulant medication such as Ritalin.

The finding of reduced white matter in the right frontal and posterior regions of the brain suggests that systems commonly associated with sustained attention are different for children with ADHD, which may help explain the difficulty these children have in more advanced attention-related functions, such as self-regulation. Reduced white matter leads to less communication between the frontal and posterior areas. The posterior region of the brain is responsible for accessing information from previous situations, while the frontal region of the brain applies this knowledge to the current situation at hand. When there is not enough communication between these two centers, the child will have difficulty either accessing previously learned information or applying it correctly to the new situation. This corresponds to the finding that children with ADHD have difficulty applying rules, even though they may be perfectly able to recite them.

What might cause ADHD? Studies suggest a potential link between cigarette-smoking and alcohol-use during pregnancy and ADHD in children. In addition, preschoolers who are exposed to high levels of lead, which can sometimes be found in plumbing fixtures or paint in old buildings, may have a higher risk of developing ADHD. Another factor might be the use of food additives such as artificial colors or preservatives. However, these findings are still rather controversial. New hypotheses pop up with alarming speed.

Another case of impaired brain development on the rise may be autism. It has been found that the brains of toddlers with autism are 10% larger than same-aged peers. Interestingly, there is no difference in head size at birth, so the brain growth that later occurs may be due to early overgrowth of neurons and a lack of synaptic pruning. Structural MRI analyses confirmed this and revealed smaller amounts of white matter (composed of nerve fibers) compared to gray matter (made up of cell bodies). Other studies of adults with autism used PET scans and found a reduced size of the structure that connects the two hemispheres, as well as difficulties with inter-regional integration, which is also a white-matter function.

What could be the cause of autism? It should be admitted that we do not really know. Some theories link autism to vaccines, but the medical community has soundly refuted these theories, although a very passionate group of parents continues to disagree. There is some evidence that autism is linked to problems in the immune system, as autistic individuals often have other physical issues related to immune deficiency. This may also explain the connection with vitamin-D deficiency. Animal studies have repeatedly shown that severe vitamin-D deficiency during gestation leads to rat pups with increased brain size and enlarged ventricles, abnormalities similar to those found in autistic children. Falling vitamin-D levels over the last 20 years due to sun-avoidance may explain autism's rapid increase in incidence during that time. The very different effects estrogen and testosterone have on vitamin D metabolism may explain why boys are much more likely to get autism than girls.

Lower vitamin-D levels in blacks may explain their higher rates of autism. However, the evidence is not yet strong enough to show a clear causal relationship.

In general, we must come to the conclusion that autism is a quite complex disorder. The range of symptoms is so varied that it probably is a catch-all term to describe a collection of related disorders. The genetic research on it is quite good, but also points to a very complex interaction of numerous variants in a variety of genes. Vitamin-D deficiency may be one of many possible environmental triggers. Clearly much more research needs to be done.

Sexual Differentiation

In the previous section, we talked about differences between males and females. How would these affect brain development? As a matter of fact, the development of the brain does vary between males and females; they mature at different times and in different ways.

Neuroscientists have known for many years that the brains of men and women are not identical. Men's brains tend to be more lateralized—that is, the two hemispheres operate more independently during specific mental tasks like speaking or navigating one's environment. For the same kinds of tasks, females tend to use both of their cerebral hemispheres more equally. So males seem to have more front-back brain connections, whereas females have more side-side connections. Another difference is brain size. Males of all ages tend to have slightly larger brains, on average, than females, even after correcting for differences in body size.

Electrical measurements have also revealed differences in boys' and girls' brain functions from the moment of birth. By three months of age, their brains respond differently to the sound of human speech. Because they appear so early in life, such differences are presumably a product of sex-related genes or hormones. We do know, though, that testosterone levels rise in male fetuses as early as seven weeks of gestation, and that this hormone affects the growth and survival of neurons in many parts of the brain. Female sex hormones may also play a role in shaping brain development, but their function is still not well understood.

Sex differences in the brain are also reflected in the somewhat different developmental timetables of girls and boys. Female infants are slightly more advanced when it comes to vision, hearing, memory, smell, and touch. Female babies also tend to be somewhat more socially attuned—responding more readily to human voices or faces, or crying more vigorously in response to another infant's cry—and they generally are ahead of boys in the emergence of fine motor and language skills.

Boys eventually catch up in many of these areas. By age three, they tend to out-perform girls in one cognitive area: visual-spatial integration, which is involved in navigation, assembling jigsaw puzzles, and certain types of hand-eye coordination. Males tend to perform better than females when it comes to tasks like mental rotation (imagining how a particular object would look if it were turned by ninety degrees), whereas females of all ages tend to perform better than males at certain verbal tasks and at identifying emotional expression in another person's face. One word of caution: while it can be helpful for parents and teachers to understand the different tendencies of the two sexes, they should not expect all children to conform to these norms.

As discussed earlier, the absence or presence of a Y-chromosome does lead to a sexual difference, but we should not confuse a difference in *sex*—such as producing either sperm cells or egg cells—with a difference in *gender*. A difference in gender entails much more than just a difference in biological characteristics—namely, differences in behavioral traits, social roles, and cultural expectations that come with being a man or a woman. "Male" and "female" are sex categories, while "masculine" and "feminine" are gender categories. Very early in a child's development, parents as well as society take on a molding role. As soon as parents know their child is a boy, for instance, they tend to treat it as a boy, which makes the child consider himself as of the male gender—and the same goes for girls. This may partly explain why girls can differ in femininity and boys in masculinity.

So it is questionable whether differences in gender are only the outcome of differences in sex, which in turn are supposedly based on differences in genes. Whereas sex differences are "in-born," gender differences appear to be more imprinted or even "self-taught."

When we talk about homosexuality, for example, we are talking in terms of gender. Homosexuality is not a change in sex—of producing either egg cells or sperm cells—but rather a matter of gender, which suggests it is many steps away from the genotype, and hence, allows for many inroads from the environment as well.

Puberty

The differences between the two sexes become more prominent when puberty sets in. Puberty is a period of several years in which rapid physical growth and psychological changes occur, culminating in sexual maturity. The average onset of puberty is at age 10 or 11 for girls and age 12 or 13 for boys—but now there seems to be a trend towards an even earlier start.

Puberty begins with a surge in hormone production, which in turn causes a number of physical changes. It is also the stage of life in which a child develops its so-called secondary sex characteristics—for example, a deeper voice and larger Adam's apple in boys, and development of breasts and more curved and prominent hips in girls. These changes are triggered by the pituitary gland, which secretes a surge of hormonal agents into the blood stream, initiating a chain reaction. The male and female gonads are subsequently activated, which puts them into a state of rapid growth and development; as a consequence, testosterone is released by the testes, and estrogen by the ovaries. The production of these hormones increases gradually until sexual maturation has been reached.

The major landmark of puberty for males is the first ejaculation, which occurs, on average, at age 13. For females, it is menarche, the onset of menstruation, which occurs, on average, between ages 12 and 13. The age at which menarche occurs is influenced by heredity, but a girl's diet and lifestyle contribute as well. Regardless of genes, a girl must have a certain proportion of body fat to attain menarche. Consequently, girls who have a high-fat diet and who are not physically active begin menstruating earlier, on average, than girls whose diet contains less fat and whose activities involve fat-reducing exercise. Girls who experience malnutrition or are in societies in which children are expected to perform physical labor begin menstruating at later ages.

Menstruation is a part of what is known as the menstrual cycle. Each month, one of the two ovaries releases usually one egg cell in a process called ovulation (see also Chapter 2). A woman can become pregnant if she has sexual intercourse within a day or two before or after the egg is released. Sperm can live for as long as 6 days, so if there is intercourse between 5 days before the release of the egg and 24 hours after, a sperm cell will be able to fertilize the egg.

During a few days preceding ovulation, the lining of the uterus becomes enlarged and thickened with blood in order to prepare for the possibility of fertilization. If the egg cell is not fertilized, both the egg and the lining are shed about 14 days after the beginning of ovulation. This discharge, called menstruation or a menstrual period, lasts on average five days. During the next nine days, a new lining grows in the uterus, after which the process of ovulation starts again. The entire cycle lasts on average 28 days, but this may slightly vary.

It is during the stage of puberty that the so-called primary sexual differences between males and females—vagina, ovaries and uterus for a female, penis and testes for a male—give rise to more pronounced secondary sexual differences, such as facial hair and an adam's apple for males and enlarged breasts for females. It is also during this time that gender differences may become more pronounced. Puberty is not only characterized by the development of differences in terms of sex and gender, but also by an accelerated growth of different body parts. This growth process happens at different times, but for all adolescents it has a fairly regular sequence. The first to grow are the extremities—the head, hands, and feet—followed by the arms and legs, and then the torso and shoulders. This non-uniform growth is one reason why an adolescent body may seem to be out of proportion for a while.

Another important element of puberty is the further development of the brain. During adolescence, the brain goes through even more intricate changes. Some of the most developmentally significant changes in the brain occur in the prefrontal cortex, which is involved in decision-making and cognitive control, as well as other higher cognitive functions. During adolescence, myelination and synaptic pruning in the prefrontal cortex increase, improving the efficiency of information-processing, and strengthening neural connections between the prefrontal cortex and other regions of the brain. This leads to better evaluation of risks and rewards, improved control over impulses, and better decision-making.

Adolescence is a time for rapid cognitive development. It is a stage of life in which the individual's thoughts start taking more of an abstract form, whereas egocentric thoughts decrease. This allows the individual to think and reason in a wider context, thanks to cognitive skills that enable the control and coordination of thoughts and behavior. The thoughts, ideas, and concepts developed at this period of life greatly influence one's future life, playing a major role in character and personality formation. No wonder some of us consider this period from birth to adolescence to be a major factor in shaping the rest of our lives. It is a rule of life that whatever happens in a previous stage has consequences for the next stage.

BEHIND THE BIOLOGICAL FACTS

The previous description of brain development may have created the impression that the brain works more or less like a computer. The way we talked about a network of interconnected neurons may remind you of the way a computer operates with a network of mutually connected transistors and processors. Indeed, computer terminology may help us explain, or even better understand, the working of the brain, but that is far from saying that the brain *is* a computer.

Yet such a comparison remains attractive, since the brain does seem to work in the same way as a computer operates. After all, they both use a binary code based on "ones" (1) and "zeros" (0). Neurons either do (1) or do not (0) fire an electric impulse—in the same way as transistors either do (1) or do not (0) conduct an electric current. So it looks as if the brain "thinks" like a computer "thinks." But does it really?

Is the Brain a Computer?

The analogy that interprets the mind as software for the computational hardware of our neuronal network is very popular nowadays.

It has been promoted so often that we lose sight of the fact that it is a very limited comparison. Just think of the following. We can transfer software from one computer to another, but not minds from one brain to another. We can run different programs on a single computer, but a human brain can only run one. And finally, computers can be made to operate precisely as we choose; minds cannot—except in science-fiction.

But there is a much more serious problem when we claim that the brain thinks like a computer "thinks." Whatever is going on in the brain—say, some particular thought—may very well have a material substrate that does work like a binary code, but it would not really matter whether this material substrate uses impulses, as it does in the brain, or currents, as in a computer. Apparently this material is only a physical carrier, a vehicle that carries something else—in the way trains can transport people or goods.

What is it, then, that the binary code of the brain carries when it comes to thinking? The obvious answer is: *thoughts.* One and the same thought could be coded in Morse, Braille, hieroglyphics, or any code language, even impulses. It does not really matter which kind of code is used, as these codes are just physical carriers or vehicles for something else. The medium is not the message! So it seems to be that the brain does not create thoughts but merely transports them; the thoughts somehow utilize the vehicle. The brain is a vehicle of thoughts coming from the mind in the same sense as a book or a CD can be a vehicle of thoughts created by the mind of its maker.

The idea that computers are the equivalent of human brains obscures the fact that computers always require the brains of a human being—not only to produce those machines but also to use them. Without the brains of human beings, who are their designers, computers cannot "think." Computers do not create thoughts, but they may carry thoughts that were created by the mind of a human person—for example, when using a word-processing program. Consider a voice recognition system; it does not really understand what it is programmed to "recognize." Computers only do what we, human beings with a mind, cause them to do, for we have proven to be champion machine-builders. True, a computer can be programmed to make decisions with an if-then-else structure, but this does not mean that the computer deliberates and decides—programmers did, and they make it look like the machine did.

Sure, a computer may play chess better than Kasparov or any other champion, but it plays the game for the same "reason" a calculator adds or a pump pumps—the reason being that it is a machine designed for that purpose—and not because it "wants" to or is "happy" to do so. A machine does not have an "I" behind it—other than the "I" of its maker. No matter what I think when I am thinking, it is always "I" who is thinking something. It is not the brain that does the thinking, but the "I"—that is, my mind. To use an analogy, it is not the wing that flies, but the bird.

When asking myself the question "Who am I?," I am certainly not doing so to find out my own name, gender, or age. Instead, I am searching for something "behind" these personal details—something unique that does not and cannot belong to anyone else. And yet, we cannot put our finger on what this "I" stands for. It is like my shadow—always a pace ahead of me, leaving open what the next step will be. Our identities do not change when we gain or lose a few particles from the collection of particles that make up our bodies. The atoms in each of us are being continually changed by eating and drinking, wear and tear. They in themselves cannot be the source of our experience of a continuing self. Indeed, since some of the atoms which are currently a part of me may in the future be a part of you, it is clear that these atoms cannot contain within themselves the principle of our identity. Although my body changes constantly, I myself do not—that is, my identity remains the same. In a sense, the body is something we *have*, but also something we *are*.

After these short remarks, I hope that a recognition of the fact that there is always some "I" behind all thinking silences the slogan that the brain is just a computer. We will get back to this issue later on (in Chapter 5).

Are We Pre-programmed?

The previous section may also have created another misleading impression that needs to be corrected. The development of the brain is not completely at the mercy of genes and DNA. An estimated 50% of a human's genes are believed to be involved in forming and running the central nervous system. However, at every step of brain development, genes necessarily interact with their environment, inside and outside the body. It is one's experiences after birth, rather than something innate, that determine the actual wiring of the human brain.

Generally speaking, genes probably regulate the basic wiring plan of the brain—forming all of the neurons and the general connections between different brain regions—but it is *experience* that is responsible for fine-tuning these connections, thus helping children adapt to the particular environment in which they grow up. The brain does everything that it is born to do, but it does so without knowing how to do what it is born to do—it needs experience.

Brain development is "activity-dependent," which means that the electrical activity in every circuit—sensory, motor, emotional, and cognitive—shapes the way the circuits get put together. Every experience excites certain neural circuits while leaving others inactive. Those that are consistently turned on over time will be strengthened, while those that are rarely excited may be dropped away. Use them or lose them, as they say. The environment can either increase abilities or diminish them. No wonder that a child of average capacity in an enriched environment may accomplish much more than a bright child in an impoverished environment.

Here is another example. Each one of us is born with the potential to learn a language. Our brains may very well be genetically programmed, more or less, to recognize human speech, to identify subtle differences between individual speech sounds, and to pick up the grammatical rules for ordering words in sentences. However, the particular language children master, the size of their vocabulary, and the exact dialect and accent with which they speak are determined by the social environment in which they are raised—that is, the thousands of hours spent listening and speaking to others. Genetic potential is essential, but DNA alone cannot teach a child to talk. In that sense, we are not pre-programmed.

Of course, the brain is partly determined by our DNA, but at the same time it is many steps away from DNA in the sense that there are many interfering factors that turn the brain into what it ends up being. Because the end-result, the *phenotype*, is many steps away from the *genotype*, the DNA, it thus allows for many inroads from the environment. It is due to this interaction of multiple factors— genetic as well as environmental—that we develop brains different from one another. And this process keeps progressing, as with a feedback mechanism. The brain affects our behavior, but then this behavior in turn affects the brain again. It is like an unending loop.

Even if we accept that genes affect hormones, and that hormones affect the brain, and that the brain affects our behavior, it still needs to be stressed that this behavior in turn affects the brain again. Consider a similar phenomenon in sports: strong muscles benefit those who play sports, but playing sports greatly benefits the development of muscles. In regard to environmental reinforcing conditions, consider that even simple things such as being a first or only child can make a huge difference in growing up. It has been shown that birth-order does have an impact on children's personality.

The outcome of this growth process is that adolescents end up with their very own "personal" brain makeup. Even identical twins have gone through their own individual growth processes, so they may differ dramatically in phenotype in spite of the fact that they do have the same genotype. And even if they are look-alikes (or act-alikes), those resemblances could very well be the result of their *desire* to be alike. Genetics may provide the raw brain material, but it is experience that ultimately molds the brain.

Nature or Nurture?

Is there a way to peel genetics and experience apart? This is the question of the nature-nurture debate. It is not only genes, hormones, and the brain that shape our behavior, but everything that we see and hear around us, plus all the dreams, hopes, ideals, plans, and expectations we foster in our minds. All of these have an impact on the way we develop ourselves. What seems to be "in-born" (nature) may very well be imprinted or even "self-taught" (nurture). To put it in a slogan: Nature is the genetic element, nurture the "contagious" element. If you happen to have children yourself, you are supposed to *raise* them with "good nurture"—which is more than giving them your DNA.

However, very often, or maybe even always, it is nearly impossible to tell what is due to "nature" and what is due to "nurture." Scientists have ferociously tried to peel them apart, but that is easier said than done. Numerous studies have been undertaken; the best ones are based on a combination of adoption research and twin research—identical twins split by adoption. But even those have pitfalls.

Adoption research on its own is not good enough. Although it is clear that relatives resemble each other more than strangers—because they have more alleles in common—it is also obvious that parents not only give alleles to their children but also parts of their environment. Even adopted children did share, for at least nine months, the surroundings of their mother's womb, including her voice, her hormones, her food, her drinks, her moods, and even her medications. Furthermore, adoption often takes place in an environment that is very similar to the original one, often just around the block or with relatives or friends. As a consequence, we tend to *over*-estimate the impact genes have if we go by adoption research alone.

On the other hand, twin research, on its own, is not good enough either. Identical twins have the same alleles, but that does not mean they are genetically identical; differences have been found in twins' DNA, especially in its non-coding parts. Besides, twins' similarities are the result not only of identical alleles but also of almost identical surroundings—at least the same womb, that is, and often the same placenta, to which both are exposed even if they end up being adopted. Their strong resemblance also makes it more likely that they will be treated by others in the same way later on in life, which may make them desire even more to be like one another. So in this case we would again *over*-estimate the impact of genes.

As a consequence, in considering the results of twin research or adoption research we tend to underestimate the "nurture" component. Another complication is the fact that twin and adoption studies often yield different estimates of the genetic component. Combining them is perhaps the best way there is to correct for the fact that they are rather skewed on their own.

Another problem with this kind of research is that we need samples that are not biased but represent the total population accurately. In one case, for instance, scientists studied members of an organization of male homosexuals and found that they had come from families with a significantly higher percentage of male siblings—whatever that means. What they did not realize, though, is that families with only female offspring were not represented in their sample at all, and thus they were under-represented in proportion to the percentage of female siblings in other families. To correct for this inherent sampling error in a statistically correct manner is extremely complicated.

What seems to be clear in all of this, however, is that while genes and hormones do set the ball rolling, they do not fully account for something like sex differences in children's brains. Experience certainly plays a fundamental role here. Consider, for example, the "typical" boy, with his more advanced spatial skills; he may well prefer activities like climbing or pushing trucks around—all of which further sharpen his visual-spatial skills. The "typical" girl, by contrast, may gravitate more toward games with dolls and her siblings, which further reinforce her verbal and social skills. It is not hard to see how initial strengths are thus magnified—thanks to the remarkable plasticity of young children's brains—into significant differences, even before boys and girls begin preschool.

But this remarkable plasticity also provides parents and other caregivers with a wonderful opportunity to compensate for the different tendencies expressed by boys and girls. For example, it is known that greater verbal interaction can improve young children's language skills. So the "typical boy" may especially benefit from a caregiver who engages him in lots of conversation and word-play. On the other hand, the "typical girl" may benefit more from a caregiver who also engages her in playing with jigsaw puzzles or building a block tower—activities that encourage her visual-spatial integration. The point is not to discourage children from sex-typical play, but to supplement such activities with experiences that encourage the development of a wider range of capabilities.

This takes us back to the distinction made earlier between "sex" and "gender." Making this distinction may be helpful to a certain extent but can also have a dubious side effect. Relying on the concept of gender sometimes obscures the reality of sex differences, making us believe we can manipulate things to our own liking. It has given certain activist movements an excuse to reject the binary division of persons into two sexes, so they can claim the freedom to be either, both, or neither, depending on their mood. However, gender does not replace sex. Male and female roles certainly have a social and cultural component, but they still reflect inherent biological differences. When a baby is born, the obstetrician or midwife announces, "It's a boy," or "It's a girl." So gender is not the sex a person decides to identify with, but rather a further development of the finer details of a person's given sex and personality. It allows for a broader scale, albeit within the dichotomy of two sexes. The gender of members of the female sex can be more or less feminine, and the gender of those of the male sex can be more or less masculine.

So it is only in a narrow and specific sense that the "gender theory" seems right. According to the World Health Organization, sex refers to the biological and physiological characteristics that define men and women, whereas gender refers to the socially constructed roles, behaviors, activities, and attributes that a given society considers appropriate for men and women. Yet this distinction may easily lead to the conclusion that a gender difference is due to nurture, and a sex difference is due to nature. However, behavior is never either all nature or all nurture, but always a very complex interweaving of both. So it is hard to keep this distinction rigidly, as is done in extreme versions of the "gender theory" which essentially claim that "gender is merely a social construction." Nonetheless, such extreme forms are not the essence of the concept of gender. At its most basic level gender theory is simply the assertion that "sex" and "gender" are not identical.

Unfortunately, the gender theory may easily turn into a gender *ideology*. When this happens, it destroys a person's identity as a man or woman. There are "gender ideologists" who want us to believe that we are not born as "F" or "M" but "X," so we can then later decide whether we want to be "F" or "M" or anything in-between. But persons whose biological sex is male cannot have a female gender identity; if they think they do, it is only in their minds as an imitation of the other sex, for whatever reason. *Sexual* orientation is not a social construction but a biological one. Yet some people in the medical field have constructed out of the blue a syndrome they call a "gender identity disorder." Labels like these are presumptuous; they tend to give questionable ideas the allure of objectivity and reality. It is this gender ideology that makes some believe that same-sex relationships are "natural"; yet the reality of the two sexes makes them realize that reproduction still requires a person of the other sex, even if that can only be "for rent."

In 2012, Pope Emeritus Benedict XVI addressed this issue, connecting an extreme version of the gender theory with the words of Simone de Beauvoir: "One is not born a woman, one becomes so." The pontiff declared the term "gender," when taken this way, to represent a new philosophy of sexuality: "According to this philosophy, sex is no longer a given element of nature, that man has to accept and personally make sense of: it is a social role that we choose for ourselves, while in the past it was chosen for us by society." It basically confuses sex with gender, and thus confuses sexual identity with gender identity. Boston College philosopher Peter Kreeft seems to be right on target when he remarked that the words *masculinity* and *femininity* "have been reduced from archetypes to stereotypes.... The main fault in the old stereotypes was their too-tight connection between sexual being and social doing, their tying of sexual identity to social roles, especially for women: the feeling that it was somehow unfeminine to be a doctor, lawyer, or politician. But the antidote to this illness is not confusing sexual identities but locating them in our being rather than in our doing." Masculinity and femininity are complementary—different but equal expressions of what it is to be human.

Sexual identity refers to *being* male or female; it refers to the specific sex of the human person. For example, men simply cannot, as males, bear or gestate children, as they do not have such a potency; but women can. Thus, being male or female is essential to who and what a person is. Gender, on the other hand, refers to certain emotional dispositions or traits characteristic of femininity or masculinity. Once we understand this distinction, sex cannot be changed. We are either male or female persons, and nothing can change that. A person's body is a fundamental indication of which sex he or she belongs to. It is a physical, empirically verifiable reality that does not change simply because our beliefs or desires do. A person can mutilate his or her genitals, but cannot change his or her sex. A person can change their genitalia, but not their sex.

Receiving hormones of the opposite sex and removing genitalia are not sufficient to change one's sex. After commissioning a study of the outcomes of sex-change operations, Dr. Paul McHugh, in his capacity as chair of the Department of Psychiatry, put a stop to gender reassignment surgery at Johns Hopkins Hospital. He wrote: "We psychiatrists, I thought, would do better to concentrate on trying to fix their minds and not their genitalia." The physician Carl Elliott once remarked that cultural and historical conditions have not just revealed transsexuals but may actually be creating them. This may explain why so-called gender-identity disorder is on the rise; it seems to have become contagious. Because of an increasing number of broken families and same-sex parents, a child may not have the right parent to identify with, and therefore its gender may not have a chance to line up with the appropriate sex. As noted by Joseph Backholm, "The irony is that a sex change itself reinforces the gender stereotypes they claim to be rejecting."

Trans-sexual individuals could in fact be compared to trans-racial individuals. There are many similarities. In either case, it is a *decision* to transition. Consider the recent case of someone who claimed a "transracial identity," in a way similar to claims of a transsexual identity. This sparked a conversation that we didn't even know we needed to have. As hard as it is to change one's sex, it is equally hard to change one's race. You do not change your race from white to black, or vice versa, by merely wishing to do so. Is it really possible for an individual to be born "in the wrong skin"? Even if it is possible, it is hard to see how it can be changed. Even if you identify closely with the black community, that does not make you black. Something similar could be said about transsexual or transgender individuals. In either case, proponents of transition are quick to claim they want to redefine "traditional labels" of sexuality, and now of ethnicity. Yet perception does not change reality. Transgendered men do not become women, nor do transgendered women become men. And something similar holds for transracial individuals—they do not become members of another race. A man declaring he is a woman is just as odd as a white woman declaring she is black.

Learning Just in Time

Since the brain is a work in progress, we should always keep in mind that *educational* goals have to stay in sync with the *biological* development of the brain. I remember from my own experience that it took me a few extra months to grasp grammatical points in Latin during my first year in middle school, and that it took me a few more months at the end of middle school to understand a concept as abstract as "institution." Perhaps I was a few months behind biologically, or the curriculum was a few months ahead of the proper time (I tend to think the latter, of course). Even some adults still find it hard to distinguish between the church as a building and the Church as a Catholic institution.

Because the brain goes through dramatic changes, adolescents have a way of behaving and thinking that is rather different from that of children during previous stages of development. Adolescents' thinking is less bound to concrete events than that of children; they can contemplate possibilities outside the realm of what currently exists, because of their improved skills in deductive reasoning, which in turn lead to the development of hypothetical thinking. This provides the ability to plan ahead, see future consequences of an action, and provide alternative explanations of events. It also makes adolescents more skilled debaters, as they can reason against a friend's or parent's assumptions.

The appearance of more systematic, abstract thinking is a striking aspect of cognitive development during adolescence. For example, adolescents find it easier than children to comprehend the higher-order abstract logic inherent in puns, proverbs, metaphors, and analogies. Their increased facility permits them to appreciate the ways in which language can be used to convey multiple messages, such as pun, satire, metaphor, and sarcasm. This also permits the application of advanced reasoning and logical processes to social and ideological matters such as interpersonal relationships, politics, philosophy, religion, morality, friendship, faith, democracy, fairness, and honesty.

Adolescents are now more able to conceptualize a variety of "possible selves" they could become, as well as long-term possibilities and consequences of their choices. Exploring these possibilities may result in abrupt changes in self-presentation as adolescents choose or reject certain qualities and behaviors, trying to guide their actual self toward the self they wish to be, and away from the self they do not wish to be. Obviously, the actual course of this process depends largely on the "quality" of their home base, circle of peers, and repertoire of role models. Eventually, though, adolescents will find their own identity, which represents a coherent sense of self that is stable across circumstances, including past experiences and future goals.

It is very evident from all of this that education can play a vital role during this growing-up process. However, we should not take "education" in a purely cognitive sense. Education is first of all the formation of character, as Herbert Spencer used to say. In 1925, the U.S. Supreme Court heard a case that is commonly known as the Oregon School case, in which the justices declared unconstitutional a state law mandating education in public schools, stating that "The child is not the mere creature of the state; those who nurture him and direct his destiny have the right, coupled with the high duty, to recognize and prepare him for additional obligation." This opened the door for private, non-public schools.

With this Supreme Court decision, the freedom of parents to choose their children's education was guaranteed throughout the United States. The idea that schools should not only prepare students for careers but also help shape character is an idea that extends back to the ancient Greeks. This should not be confused with indoctrination. If one believes that children have more than a biological dimension, then omitting other dimensions from education is itself indoctrination of another kind. It is our duty to give our children the education that we consider best, and this includes religious education. We shouldn't be fooled by the slogan that tells us children ought to make such choices on their own. After all, parents did not let them choose whether they wanted to be born; parents even decided on their names and many other things.

Character formation may certainly take place in school, but it begins in the family. We cannot expect schools to correct what goes wrong in the family. The family is of vital importance in the development of human beings. Babies can tell their mother from their father as early as six weeks—sometimes even three—after birth. Almost invariably, having made this distinction they become calm in the presence of the mother and aroused and stimulated by the approach of the father. The interactions between infant and father, as between infant and mother, have effects on both and follow a pattern that transcends social class and cultural expectations. Children whose fathers help care for them have been shown to be less likely to become violent; they have higher IQs, better impulse control, and better social adaptations—in short, better psychological health. And as for fathers themselves, studies of inner-city men have shown that fathers who help care for their children also learn from this experience and are less prone to commit crimes or join gangs.

The family is the cornerstone of society. *The Catechism of the Catholic Church* (2207) calls the family "the original cell of social life." As the philosopher Peter Kreeft notes, societies have survived with very bad political systems and very bad economies, but not without strong families. Families are grounded in the rights and duties of a marriage: Only if you marry me and stand by me can you count on me to bear and help raise your children. This requires a commitment on both sides. There is no involvement without commitment. Families are to society what cells are to a body. The family is the first place where children learn life's most important lessons, the first place where children find protection and learn the role of being a male or female. None of these "lessons" are inborn; they must be taught and nurtured! Pope Emeritus Benedict XVI stressed that within the family exists "the authentic setting in which to hand on the blueprint of human existence. This is something we learn by living it with others and suffering it with others."

There is indeed strong scientific evidence that children who spend their childhood years with their married biological parents have fewer cognitive, behavioral, and emotional problems than children who did not. Too many children grow up with an absent parent. Do not take this the wrong way: there are perfectly good single parents who raise perfectly fine children. Yet we should not forget that one of the best predictors of poverty is a broken family life.

It is usually in the family that children learn what is right and wrong—and this process begins at a very simple level. Rushing to the crib every time a child cries may train them to expect instant gratification. Children who do not learn the meaning of the word "no" will be at the mercy of impulses and desires they do not know how to control. They turn into spoiled and demanding little tyrants who cannot accept that there is a higher authority you just do not question. They have not learned the meaning of restraint. They have not been disciplined. The word "discipline" sounds rigid, and may remind some of spanking. But there is a humane alternative to spanking kids—grounding them with *timeouts*; soon even the threat of a timeout becomes effective, if followed by an explanation of why their behavior was bad. Needless to say, such an explanation only makes sense if it is in sync with the child's brain development.

Just as children learn to imitate language and gestures, they also mimic the moral practices they see at home. *The Catechism of the Catholic Church* (2207) calls the family "the community in which, from childhood, one can learn moral values, begin to honor God, and make good use of freedom." The popular saying, garbage in, garbage out, applies even here—and might also apply to what happens in dysfunctional families. Children do need and deserve a functional family. Good role models are essential, making every day a "school day" when it comes to moral development. Children who have never learned to be ashamed of certain behaviors are in real trouble, perhaps even for the rest of their lives.

This also holds for teaching teenagers about sexual matters. An important part of character formation is learning how to navigate through the tumultuous stage of puberty. Let me illustrate this for one of the two sexes in particular—the fair sex—by following the thoughts of the writer Emily Stimpson. A beautiful girl is a woman who is lovely in body and soul. Her loveliness starts on the inside and is reflected on the outside. Her beauty is about much more than the sum of her parts, so she chooses to *veil* some of her parts. Is that not what Eve's fig leaves were all about? They were intended to help

Adam see her as a subject, not an object; they were intended to protect her from being used.

True, character formation unfolds at home, but home is surrounded by a specific society and culture. The latter are telling us nowadays that being "sexy" should become the goal for the female gender in a modern society like ours. Women are being forced to think that being sexy and being beautiful are the same thing—but they are not. They actually have the opposite effect: "sexy" unveils all that beauty veils. It puts everything on display like an object in a store window. It changes subjects into objects.

Some have argued that this new trend is connected to the "sexual revolution" that can probably be traced back to Sigmund Freud and has been aimed at liberating humanity from any sexual restraints. As a consequence, we have become a culture ruled by Viagra, pornography, sexual abuse, and rape. As Peter Kreeft points out, this so-called "revolution" has only led to growing numbers of children who are sexually abused and of women who are beaten, abandoned, or raped by men who do not want to hear about self-control and consider every subject they meet a mere object ready to be (ab)used.

It needs to be confirmed once again that sex belongs to the domain of marriage, monogamy, and fidelity; that sex is for life, not only for fun; that taming the sex drive and harnessing it to the family are a necessary condition for social stability and long-term human happiness. As long as society keeps telling parents, and parents keep showing their teenage daughters and friends, that there is no difference between being sexy and being beautiful, the character formation of our next generation will be in jeopardy. And, of course, there is a similar story for the macho image of teenage boys. As stated earlier, each stage of life's journey leaves its imprint on the subsequent stages.

Another often-overlooked intruder in this process of navigating through puberty is the "magnetic tube." Of all the challenges a developing teenager faces, few are more problematic than the one we willingly bring into our homes—the television. It can be a blessing on certain occasions, but it also comes in with its own ulterior motives. It captivates teenagers, sometimes when parents cannot, and it teaches them things parents would not. The problem with TV is just what is it teaching our children, even when it is presumably "educational"? The commercial networks go for where the money is—adolescents. The hand that rocks the cradle may rule the world, but the hand that holds the remote may become even more important.

It is clear that growing up is not just a biological process but also a development in other areas of life. One such area we have not yet considered is religion. Some parents think that children should only later, on their own, decide which religion they want, so they decide to bring up their children without any form of religion. Strangely enough, they don't let their children choose whether they want to be born, whether they want to be fed, or whether they want to go to school. Part of parenting is giving our children the best we have been given or discovered ourselves—the best food, the best education, and also the best religion. Keeping such things away from them would make them "undernourished." There are sins of omission that will haunt us until the end of our lives.

In short, while children are still in a process of growth and development, it is the parents' responsibility to feed their bodies with the right nutrition and to feed their minds with the right spiritual food. According to *The Catechism of the Catholic Church* (2252), parents "have the duty to provide as far as possible for the physical and spiritual needs of their children." Let me end this section with another reference to the sentence that begins Tolstoy's *Anna Karenina*: "Happy families are all alike; every unhappy family is unhappy in its own way."

4

Growing in Maturity

THE BIOLOGY BEHIND IT

When adolescence is over, we call ourselves "grown-ups," as though we are biologically finished and complete. The truth is far from that! Indeed, there are certain aspects of the development of brain structure and function that do level off at the end of adolescence; but the brain remains a work-in-progress, even during adulthood.

A Work-in-Progress

Although some 100 billion neurons are added during the first five months of pregnancy, and even though the number of neurons peaks just before birth, after that new neurons can still be produced throughout life, albeit far less rapidly, and probably in numbers sufficient only to replace those that gradually die off. This was not known until rather recently. Besides, as we discussed earlier, myelination is a highly extended process. Although most areas of the brain begin adding this critical insulation within the first two years of life, some of the more complex areas in the frontal and temporal lobes continue that process throughout childhood and perhaps well into a person's twenties. In particular, those critical parts of the brain involved in decision-making are not fully developed until years later—around age 25. The prefrontal cortex—which is the part of the brain that helps you to inhibit impulses and to plan and organize your behavior to reach a goal—is not yet fully developed. Under most laws, young people may be recognized as adults at age 18, but emerging science about brain development suggests that most people do not reach full maturity until the age of 25. And even then, just what is "full"?

There is no specific age at which the adolescent brain becomes an

83

adult brain. Structures responsible for logical reasoning mature by the age of 16, but those involved in self-regulation are still developing in young adulthood. This is why 16-year-olds are just as competent as adults when it comes to granting informed medical consent, but still immature in ways that diminish their criminal responsibility, as the Supreme Court has noted in several recent cases. Using different ages for different legal boundaries may seem odd, but it would make some neuro-scientific sense. However, the reality is that age boundaries are drawn for mainly political reasons, not scientific ones.

Even in adulthood, the brain is constantly remodeling itself and continuing to develop connections—yet with two major differences. First, the rate of synapse formation is much slower than in previous stages. Second, synapses are formed based only on specific experiences during the adult's life. For example, adults who witness a catastrophic event—such as the collapse of the World Trade Center in New York City—form connections in the brain that allow them to remember and process what they saw. Adults who were not there but watched news coverage of the attacks formed different networks of connections that help them remember what they saw and heard on the news.

Here we have those "experiences" again. They even play a critical role in *adult* learning. So the question is: Does the learning process undergo age-related change when adolescents become adults? The answer is that adults learn in different ways from children. Children are sponges. Every day is a new adventure in which new things are learned. But this all changes somewhere along the way when we mature and become adults. Adults only learn what they feel they need to learn.

Adult learning tends to be very practical. If adults cannot see how a given learning process will help them immediately, then the true understanding and retention rate will be very low. Adult learners can also be hindered by their greater life-experience, which tends to cause them to have more fixed cognitive patterns; for this reason they can be less open-minded than children. Children, with less life-experience, are often more open to learning new things. And yet we do speak of "continuing education"—even, or especially, for adults.

Continuing Education

For adults, the most important trait for the brain to possess is—again—plasticity. Plasticity is the ability of the brain to adapt in response to new experiences. During the first years after birth, humans manufacture an estimated 250,000 neurons per minute and then spend the next few years wiring them together. Traditionally, it was assumed that this neural plasticity settles down by adulthood; but new research has revealed that in fact it never completely disappears.

Brain plasticity allows adults to keep learning from new experiences, which they often in fact must do—when, for instance, they go back to school, expect their first baby at a later age, lose a loved one, go through a career-change, or plan to retire. At such moments, brain plasticity is in high demand—and, lo and behold, it is still there! This is also one of the reasons why humans can adapt to extreme living circumstances that confront them with incredible challenges, even at a later age: we can adapt to snorkeling in the water, learning to drive a car or fly a plane, moving to another country and culture, hiking in the Himalayas—even migrating and adjusting to a new life in a place such as New York City! As a matter of fact, plasticity of the brain has allowed humans who lost their arms in combat or accidents to adapt to using a prosthesis, even to writing with their feet.

Neuroscientists have known for decades that adult neurons can change their firing pattern and responses when faced with new experiences, but now there is evidence that neurons can also structurally change—especially a group of inhibitory neurons called "interneurons," which delay or block signals from excitatory neurons. Approximately 20–30% of the neurons in the neo-cortex, the part of the brain responsible for higher functions such as thinking, are made up of inhibitory interneurons, which play an important role in regulating brain activity by providing stop signals for excitation. This new discovery means that we can do as many healthy "workouts" for our brains as we do for our bodies.

Since lifelong activity is important to maintain healthy brain growth, areas of the brain that are not used regularly may eventually deteriorate. Keeping the mind active is a key way to prevent brain atrophy. "Activity" can be as simple as reading a book like this one, or magazines and newspapers, solving crossword puzzles, or spending time talking to others and maintaining relationships. People who isolate and dull themselves actually stop having experiences that keep the brain active—they put themselves in bad company, so to speak.

By creating new neuronal connections, the mind seems to be able to install new "programs" in the brain. Through goal-setting, self-talk (affirmations), self-examination (evaluations), and mental imagery (visualization), the mind can create new connections in the brain. Although there is much more empirical testing needed in this respect, there are strong indications as to what mental training can do for the brain, similar to what physical training does for the body. This is what some call "mind over matter."

You have heard the saying, "You can't teach an old dog new tricks"; this saying may be applicable to dogs, but not to human beings, since humans do have a capacity to continue learning throughout their entire life—which is called "continuing education." Whereas the ability of abstract reasoning does reach its full development in the late teens and starts to decline in the twenties, there is also a so-called crystallized intelligence, which is more dependent on education and cultural background, and continues to increase until the end of one's life. Middle-aged people can still learn new things, new facts and skills. Longitudinal studies have shown that IQ increases until the age of 50, and there is no evidence for a decline of intellectual functioning of adults until the age of 60. Generally the highest outcome and productivity rate is found between the ages of 40 and 70.

Malcolm Knowles introduced the concept of andragogy—meaning "the art and science of helping adults learn"—in addition to pedagogy—"the art and science of helping children learn" in order to highlight the significant differences between adult learners and learners under the age of 18. Primarily, the differences relate to an adult learner being more self-directing, having a repertoire of experience, and being internally motivated to learn subject matter that can be applied immediately—a kind of learning that is closely related to the developmental tasks of his or her social role.

Going back to Piaget's four stages of cognitive development, some have suggested there should be a fifth stage for adults: a stage of problem-*finding*, which means problem-discovery, after the fourth stage of problem-*solving*. This requires intellectual vision and insight into what is missing; it involves the application of creativity. As the philosopher John Dewey put it, "A problem is half-solved if properly stated." Whatever this thought is worth, it is an interesting and challenging idea. It may even start a remodeling process of the brain.

Menopause

During mid-life, women have to deal with a change in their reproductive capacity with which men are unfamiliar. Men continue to make sperm and testosterone at virtually the same rates, although there is some decline in testosterone levels as they age. Lower levels would cause the hypothalamus and pituitary gland to trigger a release of gonadotropin-releasing hormone (GnRH) and luteinizing hormone (LH), but this does not happen when men age. Low GnRH, low LH, and low testosterone indicate what is called hypogonadotropic hypogonadism. Eventually, testosterone levels can drop to such low levels that the hypothalamus and pituitary gland kick in and produce high levels of GnRH and LH to compensate. This triggers the production of testosterone, which will generally work for a while but then fall again. That is when men enter a period that some call "andropause." They have low testosterone and high LH- and GnRH-levels, whereas before they had a low level of testosterone as well as a low level of LH and GnRH.

Women, on the other hand, go through a much more dramatic change in their reproductive capacity. But no matter what, the menopause transition, and the time following it, is a natural life change, certainly not a disease or a disorder. The transition from a reproductive to a non-reproductive stage is the result of a reduced production of female hormones by the ovaries. This transition is not so much characterized by what is happening to the uterus as by what is happening to the ovaries. Even when the uterus has been removed, ovulation and the release of the sequence of reproductive hormones will continue to cycle on until menopause is reached. In contrast to this, if a woman's ovaries are removed while the uterus is left intact, she will immediately be in what is called "surgical menopause."

What is it, then, that is happening to the ovaries during this transition process? We mentioned already that women are born with all the eggs they are ever going to have; they do not make any new eggs during their lifetime. They are born with approximately 2,000,000 eggs in their ovaries, but about 11,000 of these die every month prior to puberty. As a teenager, a woman has only some 400,000 remaining eggs; and from that point on, approximately 1,000 eggs are destined to die each month. This phenomenon occurs independently of any hormone-production, birth-control pills, pregnancies, nutritional supplements, or even health or lifestyle. As Dr. Sherman J. Silber puts it: Whenever the woman runs out of her supply of eggs, the ovaries cease to make estrogen, and she goes through menopause. To reiterate: although some women go through menopause at different ages, the timing does not appear to depend upon any specific element in their lives other than the number of eggs with which they were endowed at birth. There is a wide variation in endowment of eggs from woman to woman, and this will determine whether a given woman loses her fertility as early as in her late twenties or early thirties, or will be able to have children into her mid- or even late-forties. When only 25,000 eggs remain in the ovaries, menopause will occur in approximately thirteen years.

The normal menstrual cycle is regulated by several hormones. Each month the hypothalamus, which is part of the brain, produces chemicals known as releasing factors. These pass into the pituitary gland below it and stimulate the production of pituitary hormones, such as follicle-stimulating hormone (FSH) and luteinizing hormone (LH). These, in turn, induce the ovaries to produce estradiol, testosterone, and progesterone in a cyclical pattern.

But when menopause sets in, some dramatic changes occur as well. Due to the eventual depletion of almost all of the egg-cell-containing follicles in the ovaries, there is a decrease in the levels of circulating follicle-stimulating hormone (FSH) and luteinizing hormone (LH) because fewer and fewer follicles respond to these hormones, and thus less and less estrogen is produced. It is this decrease in the production of estrogen that leads to the menopausal symptoms of hot flashes, insomnia, and mood changes.

When menopause sets in, the production of estrogen and progesterone by the ovaries becomes more irregular, often with wide and unpredictable fluctuations in levels. Initially, there are clear and often dramatic fluctuations in FSH and estradiol levels, which gradually end with a dramatic fall in circulating estradiol levels. In contrast to the marked fall in estradiol during menopause, the levels of total and free testosterone appear to decline more or less steadily with age, unless the ovaries are surgically removed or damaged by chemotherapy or radiotherapy.

The term "menopause" is often used in a broader sense, however, to mean the months or even years before and after this natural event in a woman's life. In the years leading up to menopause, the menstrual cycle is more jumbled and menstrual periods may become irregular. The first evidence of the onset of the menopause transition-time is the occurrence of slight variations in the *length* of the menstrual cycle. But these variations become more pronounced over time, and eventually lead to phenomena such as cycles that can be considerably longer or considerably shorter than usual, a flow that can be significantly lighter or heavier than usual, missed ovulations and menstrual periods, or spans of time of many months with no flow at all, after which menstruation may resume. The transition is considered to be complete once a woman has experienced twelve months without any menstrual bleeding at all. At this point, a woman is deemed to be a year into post-menopause, is considered infertile, and no longer must consider the possibility of becoming pregnant.

About 25% of women do not notice any changes during menopause, except for the termination of periods. Some 50% of them notice slight physical and/or mental changes. The remaining 25% experience inconvenient or even distressing symptoms. Physical symptoms may include hot flashes, dryness of the vagina, heart palpitations, and headaches. The non-physical symptoms may include anxiety, depression, trouble concentrating, and sleeping difficulties. These symptoms may last from only a few weeks to five years or more. An additional complication for one in five women is the development of osteoporosis, which may eventually lead to compression of the spine and bone structures. A diet rich in calcium is the best protection against osteoporosis.

Some women experience such severe hot flashes, night sweats, mood issues, or vaginal dryness that they consider hormone replacement therapy (HRT). This therapy consists of a treatment with estrogen, sometimes combined with progesterone. The dosage can even be varied cyclically to more closely mimic the ovarian hormone cycle, with estrogen taken daily and progesterone taken for about two weeks every month or two. However, for women who had a hysterectomy, progesterone should not be administered, and for women who no longer have a uterus, progesterone is not needed. On the other hand, women who still have a uterus do need to take progesterone in addition to estrogen to protect against the development of endometrial carcinoma.

When taking progesterone during HRT, it should be noted that oral administration may be convenient, but the oral form is rapidly metabolized and deactivated in the liver; and therefore high doses must be administered to achieve adequate circulating blood levels. To overcome this problem, synthetic progestin has been developed. This synthetic equivalent is more resistant to liver metabolism, so lower doses are needed to achieve the desired endometrial effect.

When it comes to HRT, the therapy or treatment should not be used for more than five years, as there are some health risks involved. Women who decide to use hormone replacement therapy are generally well-advised to take the lowest effective dose of hormones for the shortest period of time possible. The dangers of long-term treatment seem to be greater than the potential benefits. To reduce the risks of estrogen therapy, it may be prudent to use not an estrogen pill, but rather skin patches, IUDs, vaginal creams, vaginal rings, gels, etc.

One more word of caution: a few years ago, the American National Institute of Health declared that HRT treatment has been associated with an increased incidence of breast cancer, heart attacks, and strokes—which statement lead to a sharp decline in HRT prescription throughout the world and was soon followed by a decrease in breast cancer incidence. On the other hand, it might simply be that timing is of the essence: giving estrogen within a year or two of menopause has beneficial effects, but giving estrogen to women more than five years beyond their menopause can actually be harmful. When the women close to menopause were looked at separately, there were no adverse effects on the heart, and in fact there was some indication of beneficial effects.

Fortunately, hormones are not always needed to reduce symptoms of menopause. Because estrogen may increase the risks of breast cancer, heart attacks, and strokes, it might be wise to consider alternatives to hormone therapy. One of these options is using medicines such as antidepressants, which help with mood swings, hot flashes, and other symptoms. A healthier option might be diet and lifestyle changes: avoiding caffeine, alcohol, and spicy foods; eating foods with soy as an alternative to estrogen; or using over-the-counter plant estrogen (phyto-estrogen) and herbal remedies. This may be worth trying, as women are dealing here with an important stage in their lives—a stage that deserves adequate attention.

BEHIND THE BIOLOGICAL FACTS

Much of the growing process human beings go through seems to be under genetic control—certainly not exclusively, as we found out, but at least to a certain degree. It should not surprise us, then, that some geneticists have been obsessed with the power of genes. Often we hear or read about "a gene for intelligence," "a gene for alcoholism," "a gene for pedophilia," "a gene for bullying," "a gene for hypochondriasis," "a gene for compulsive buying"—and the list goes on and on! What do such claims mean?

In general, geneticists try to explain differences between people by differences in alleles of a specific gene. They are in search of a difference that makes a difference—that is, a difference in phenotype associated with a difference in genotype. But even then it still remains to be seen whether such a connection or association also qualifies as a *causal* relationship.

A Gene for Everything?

It is both tempting and easy to come up with a trait that distinguishes a group of people from other groups. Here follows a rather arbitrary collection of designations that lump certain people together: attention-deficit/hyperactivity disorder (ADHD), bi-sexuality, alcoholism, kleptomania, pedophilia—and all such syndromes as hypothyroid syndrome, restless leg syndrome, adrenal fatigue syndrome, gender identity disorder, Munchausen syndrome (in which people fake illness). And what to think of ODD, opposition defiant disorder? Geneticists love to identify certain similarities between people and then link them to a particular gene, claiming they have made a scientific discovery. They love to "label" and "categorize," but often without much to base it on.

To put it bluntly, not all inventions entail discoveries. The person who invented "Atlantis" did not discover Atlantis; it remains a legendary island until further notice. The same goes for science: most inventions do not entail discoveries. Yet some scientists think they have made a discovery when all they have made is an invention, a hypothesis. As a consequence, we have been bombarded with "discoveries" of new genes: a gene for longevity, a gene for homosexuality, a gene for schizophrenia, a gene for altruism, and even a gene for religion—the list could go on and on. These hypothetical genes were once claimed, and then often had to be retracted; repeatedly they were shown to be inventions rather than discoveries.

Reacting to the casual way in which some neurobiologists speak of a gene for depression or a gene for violence, one could argue that terms such as "depression" and "violence" are very simple labels for very complicated and variable patterns of behavior. They make for rather complicated phenomena that come in many varieties. Nevertheless, genetic determinism remains very rampant among scientists, so hypothetical genes just keep coming and going. That is where science approaches science fiction. One could even come up with a gene that makes one believe in the all-powerfulness of genetics!

Not all these inventions are bogus, of course, but most of them are still in the stage of hypothesis and are awaiting the stage of confirmation. And yet it remains tempting to claim a genetic cause for a "diagnosis" that may not even exist. Perhaps alcoholism is not genetic but rather something acquired at home, or in the womb, or in a group of one's peers. Perhaps pedophilia is not an issue of genetics but rather a form of immoral behavior—rape, that is. Perhaps Munchausen Syndrome is only a call for attention or sympathy. It is certainly not fair to put them all in the same category of questionable diagnoses, but it is reasonable to signal how often we get bombarded with a new "disease." First they invent a disease, then they invent the gene to explain such a disease—and then they sell us an elixir to cure it! Instead, we could very well be dealing with phantom-diseases and bogus genes. Geneticists like to invent a gene for any disease imaginable—just as hypochondriacs believe they may actually have any disease imaginable (except hypochondriasis, of course).

Let us never forget that, in addition to differences in genetic make-up, there are also personal and cultural variations. We often acquire habits at home, in school, and through peers or friends, as well as through the society we live in—such habits need not be *genetic* in origin. Things can be hereditary without being genetic. To put it differently, there certainly is not a gene for everything. If you never touch alcohol or illegal drugs, you will not develop an addiction to these substances. If you do touch them, however, it is not clear whether this is a genetic compulsion or not rather peer pressure, or an act of depression, or even mere curiosity; indeed, it could well be any of the above. Even if there is something like a genetic "predisposition," we should not forget that these so-called predispositions can often be reprogrammed.

In short, it is hard to believe there is such a thing as a "chip gene" for people with an addiction to chips, a "chocolate gene" for chocoholics, or a "spending gene" for big spenders. Genetic determinism certainly has its limitations. We are not at the mercy of our genes, and our genes are not our destiny; they are like a hand of cards we are dealt, but we can play them differently. Human behavior may be more often than not a matter of lifestyle *choices* rather than the outcome of a set of genetic instructions. The judgments that lead to choices humans make are free because humans are in control of those choices. This is why we have thieves, liars, and kidnappers; but it is also why we can have doctors, nurses, judges, and teachers. Human beings are free to choose to act or not to act. But even if there are genes that determine a certain behavior, we need to realize that genes often must be "turned on" by an outside force before they can do their "pre-programmed" job.

The outside force of high stress-levels, for instance, may activate a variety of genes, including those suspected of being involved in fear, shyness, and some mental illnesses. Children conceived during a three-month famine in the Netherlands during a Nazi blockade in 1945 were later found to have twice the rate of schizophrenia of that among Dutch children born to parents who were spared the trauma of famine. There is always more to it than merely genes. When it comes to genes, we could very well recite the phrase, "It ain't necessarily so."

Rationality and Morality

There is not a gene for everything, as we have seen, and there is certainly not a gene for rationality or morality. We are beings with a free will—free to make decisions, rational or irrational, moral or immoral. Our lives should be lived under the guidance of rationality and morality; we are endowed with the faculties of rationality and morality, which seem to set us apart from the animal world. Rationality gives us access to the world of truths and untruths—a world beyond our control; yet we have an immaterial sense for what is true and what is false. Morality gives us access to a world of duties and rights—a world also beyond our control, although we do have an immaterial sense of what is morally right and what is morally wrong. Since the above statements may raise many questions, let us discuss first what that pair of two concepts stands for, and then, later, we will learn why rationality and morality cannot have a genetic basis.

As *rational* beings, endowed with the capacity of rationality, we are in pursuit of what is *true* (versus *false*). Rationality gives us an "immaterial sense" for what is true and what is false. It is our capacity for abstract thinking and having reasons for our thoughts, thus giving us access to the "unseen" world of thoughts, laws, and truths. Rationality allows us to gain knowledge about the world through the power of abstract concepts and logical reasoning. Reasoning leads us from one idea to a related idea; it does not work with signals but with symbols; it is a matter of pondering realities beyond that which we experience through our physical senses, thus allowing us to transcend our current situation. This is very different from processing images and signals—it is about working with symbols and concepts. Weighing evidence and coming to a conclusion are rational activities par excellence.

It is rationality that makes the world intelligible; it gives us the power to understand the universe, and to maintain self-control when emotions tend to take over. Without the human mind, without its intellect and rationality, there would not even be any science—or worse, there would not even be any facts, for facts are mental interpretations of this world, made through our intellect, as discussed earlier (see Chapter 1). Animals certainly live in a world of events, but humans also inhabit a world of facts—which are mental interpretations of those events. The world of animals is only populated with what their physical senses can capture, whereas capturing facts requires a spiritual mind, with something like a sixth sense. That is where rationality comes in. Rationality makes us search for what is true and what is false. Rationality makes assessments. We are not only rational beings, but also *moral* beings. Keep in mind, though, that *morality* is not another word for social behavior. These two are very different notions. Whereas social behavior can also be found in the animal world, morality cannot. What is it, then, that makes the two so different?

Morality is unconditional. Most other rules and laws tell us what we should do in order to reach a certain goal—they are conditional means to other ends: If you want to learn, you must do this; if you want to recover from a cold, you must do so-and-so; and so on. Moral laws and rules, on the other hand, are based on absolute, universal, non-negotiable moral *values*, so they are unconditional ends-in-themselves. As C.S. Lewis once put it, "The human mind has no more power of inventing a new value than of imagining a new primary color." Morality tells us what *ought* to be done—no matter what, whether we like it or not, whether we feel it or not, or whether others enforce it or not. Moral truth is greater than man's inventions, greater than what "man" deems right and wrong at any particular time.

As moral beings, endowed with the capacity for morality, we are in pursuit of what is *right* (versus *wrong*). Not everything that is thinkable or possible or reasonable is also permissible. Morality is about our rights and obligations, about which actions others owe us and which actions we owe to others as part of the "common good." Duties and rights go hand in hand, so they have a natural reciprocity: the duty of self-preservation is also the right of self-preservation; the duty to seek the truth is also the right to seek it; the duty to work for justice is also the right to pursue it. In other words, no duties means no rights, and no rights means no duties. To give a few other examples: there is no duty to die, so there is no right to die; no duty to marry, so no right to marriage; no duty to have children, so no right to have children.

So morality is not about what the world *is* like, but about what the world *ought* to be like; it is not a matter of description but of prescription. We cannot derive moral values from the way things are; Newton's law of gravity says something about how things are, but not about how things ought to be. This has become known as the rule that "ought" cannot be derived from "is." "Racial equality," for instance, is not a descriptive term but a prescriptive one; the various human races are not equal in terms of their characteristics but they do have the same dignity and rights. Morality tells us what ought to be done—by us, as a duty, and towards us, as a right—lest a moral mistake be made. Therefore, morality is not a matter of political correctness but of moral correctness. It makes us search for what is intrinsically right and what is intrinsically wrong.

What rationality and morality have in common is that they seem to set us apart as human beings, for they are not in our DNA and therefore do not come from the animal world. That is a claim that needs further corroboration. Let us consider the case of rationality first. Rationality is not a matter of intelligence but of intellect. The main difference is that intelligence can be graded on a scale, but intellect cannot. If you want to question this distinction between intelligence and intellect, you should read the rather technical following two paragraphs—otherwise skip them.

Intelligence only works with *perception* through the senses. Many animals show some form of intelligence in their behavior, because intelligence is a brain feature and as such an important tool in survival. Animals show various forms of intelligence: we find spatial intelligence in pigeons and bats, social intelligence in wolves and monkeys, formal intelligence in apes and dolphins, and practical intelligence in rats and ravens, to name just a few. Intelligence is a matter of processing sensory data—something even a robot can do by "cleverly" processing sounds, images, patterns, and the like. All of this can be done with various degrees of accuracy and intricacy.

Intellect is very different from intelligence. Like intelligence, intellect uses sensory data, but unlike intelligence it changes perception into *cognition* by means of concepts and reasoning, thereby making sensory experiences *intelligible* for the human mind. A given concept may be as simple as a "circle" or as complex as a "gene," but any concept definitely goes beyond what the senses provide. Concepts are also very different from images. Images are by nature ambiguous, open to various interpretations; in order to interpret them we need concepts. We do not see genes but have come to hypothesize them in a concept. We do not even see circles, for a "circle" is a highly abstract, idealized concept (with a radius and diameter). Once these concepts have been established and mastered, we have become "regular observers" of "circles" and "genes." But again, these are not images but concepts.

It is through mental concepts that we transform "things" of the world into "objects" of knowledge; concepts change experiences into observations, thus enabling humans to see with their "mental eyes" what no physical eyes could ever have seen before. To be sure, all we know about the world does come through our physical senses, but this is then processed by the immaterial intellect that extracts from sensory experiences that which is *intelligible*. Obviously the intellect may aid human intelligence, but intelligence can also work on its own, as it does in animals and even robots. But the latter two do not have intellect, because they lack mental concepts and logical reasoning. You can have more or less intelligence, but you cannot have more or less intellect—humans have it, animals do not.

Let us go back to rationality. Rationality is an intellectual "tool." It gives us cognition in addition to perception; it gives us the mental power of abstract concepts and intellectual reasoning; it gives us the capacity for abstract thinking and having reasons for our thoughts, thus giving us access to the "unseen" world of thoughts, laws, and truths—allowing us to be masters of our own actions and experts in science. Reasoning is pondering realities beyond those which we experience through our senses. That is what we have been engaged in in this book—reasoning based on mental concepts.

Animals, on the other hand, are not rational—they may be more or less intelligent, but they are not rational beings. Pets can sometimes be "smarter" than their owners when they play a whole repertoire of tricks on their owner's emotions—but that is a matter of intelligence, not intellect. Animals do have the capacity to sense, imagine, and remember things; but they lack understanding in the sense of asking questions, formulating concepts, framing propositions, stating facts, and drawing conclusions. They show no signs of abstract reasoning or having reasons for their "thoughts" (if they have any); they do not think in terms of true and false; they do not think in terms of cause-and-effect with "if-and-only-if" logic; they are "moved" by motives, drives, instincts, and training, but not by intellectual reasons or mental concepts.

Because animals lack reason—that is, the ability to ponder realities beyond that which is experienced through the senses—they seem to live their lives entirely in the present, without having any thoughts about the past or the future—perhaps memories, but not thoughts. If animals have a pedigree, it is thanks to their owners; if they have birthdays, wish-lists, appointments, or schedules, it is because their owners create those; and if they have graves, those were dug by their owners as well. Cats or dogs have never come up with the thought of going to the pet store and buying their own food, let alone of starting their own pet store.

Fond as we are of anthropomorphism, we tend to think that animals must be like us—even with regard to rationality. But what a disparity there is between them and us! Only humans are conscious of time; we can study the past, recognize the present, and anticipate the future; we even desire to transcend time, thinking about living forever. Only humans wonder, "what caused or will cause what and why?" Only human beings have inquisitive minds asking questions such as "Where do we come from?" or "Why are we here?" Only humans have the capacity to be scholars and scientists; we can study animals but animals cannot study us—they can watch us but not analyze us. Human beings are always in search of some kind of worldview or explanation of life—which certainly goes far beyond the need for sex and food. In short, human beings are *questioning* beings; we are driven by rationality, which gives them the capacity to make rational decisions (without any guarantee, of course, that each particular decision is always rational).

The situation is similar with regard to morality. In the animal world, there is no morality. Only humans are able to curb their animal instincts and drives with morality. Morality makes us do what "by nature" we would never do. But animals do not have any moral values or laws, so they do not have to control their drives, lusts, and emotions. They just follow whatever "pops up" in their brains—and no one has the right to morally blame them. The relationship between predator and prey, for instance, has nothing to do with morality; if predators really had a conscience guided by morality, their lives would be pretty harsh. Dogs may act as if they are "caring," but they are just following their instinct, not some moral code; dogs happen to have such an instinct, whereas cats lack it, since it is not in their genes.

As a consequence, animals never do awful things out of meanness or cruelty, for the simple reason that they have no morality—and thus no cruelty or meanness. Humans, on the other hand, definitely do have the capacity to perform real atrocities. Animals do not; if animals do seem to do awful things, it is only because we as human beings consider their actions "awful" according to our standards of morality. Yet we will never arrange court sessions for grizzly bears that maul hikers, because we do know that bears are not morally responsible for their actions.

Since animals do exhibit social behavior but have no moral values, they have no duties, no responsibilities, and consequently no rights. If animals had rights, their fellow animals also would need to respect those. Being prone to anthropomorphism, we may assume they have morality, but they do not. Yet there is another side to the story. Since *we* do have morality, we need to treat animals, God's other creatures, humanely and responsibly—not because animals deserve it, but because humans owe it to their Maker and to themselves, being stewards of what the Maker created. Although animals are not human, we are; so we ought to treat them humanely. As Antoine de Saint-Exupéry wrote in *The Little Prince*, "You are responsible forever for that which you have tamed."

What Makes Us Rational and Moral Beings?

The question emerges, then, as to where rationality and morality come from. Although they do not seem to come from the animal world, they could still be a product of our—human—genes. But there are some serious doubts about this possibility. Let us discuss this problem first with regards to rationality.

If rationality were really a matter of genes, it would belong to the material world and would therefore be as fragile as the material world itself. It would be sitting on a swamp of molecules, unable to pull itself up by its bootstraps—which would be like an electric generator running on its own power. If rationality were really a matter of DNA, it would lose all its power. Claims can be true or false, but molecules such as DNA cannot be true or false. In order for us to make any rational claims, we need to validate our claims as being true; otherwise, they are worth nothing. If Watson and Crick were nothing but DNA, then Watson and Crick's theories about DNA must be as fragile as their DNA. That would be detrimental for their claims. If we were to claim that we are nothing but DNA, this very statement would not be worth more than its molecular origin, and neither would we ourselves who are making such a statement. The British biologist J.B.S. Haldane made this argument already some time ago, echoed by C.S. Lewis: If I believe that my beliefs are the mere product of DNA, then I have no reason to believe my belief is true—therefore, I have no reason to believe that my beliefs are the mere product of DNA.

Beliefs like these defeat and destroy themselves. As we stated earlier, if we want to accept the reliability of our biological knowledge regarding DNA, we cannot conclude that at the same time all human knowledge is just a product of DNA. That would be "irrational" suicide! If rationality were the product of DNA, we definitely should be questioning the validity of our knowledge—which necessarily includes all the scientific knowledge we wish to claim. In short, we would have no *reason* to trust our own reasoning. That would be the end of anything we claim to be true—a thought that in fact stops all thought.

Whereas genes are material entities that can be measured, issues of truth or falsehood are immaterial. A gene cannot make something true—perhaps more or less effective, more or less successful, or the like, but never true, let alone more or less true. Truth is not under the control of genes, but quite the opposite—genes are under the control of what is true in our world, of what the cosmic design allows, which includes the laws of nature. Therefore, we have the freedom to accept or reject what is true and what is false, or change our minds as to what is true and what is false—as we see happening all the time—because truth is not determined by genes.

We would run into similar problems when it comes to morality. If morality were really a matter of genes, we should first of all question why we would need articulated moral laws and rules to reinforce what "by nature" we supposedly would or would not desire to do anyway. Apparently, moral laws and rules are necessary because our genes do *not* tell us what we ought to do. As it happens, there are only far too many people willing to break moral rules when they can get away with it. Are they really fighting their genes? Do they really have alleles that make them go against what morality tells them? That claim is hard to believe, and even harder to defend.

Take, for instance, the moral responsibility parents feel towards their underage children. Is this a natural, "instinctive" responsibility that was promoted by natural selection because it presumably improves the offspring's reproductive capacity? Obviously it is not, given the fact that far too many parents try to ignore their so-called "natural" responsibility. Or take monogamy: if we were monogamous "by nature," we would not need moral laws to protect family life. In other words, we are rather dealing here with responsibility in a *moral* sense. Moral laws are absolute; they tell us to do what our genes do *not* make us do "by nature." As mentioned earlier, they are ends-in-themselves, not means to other ends. Since moral laws are not means to other ends, they have no survival value, and therefore cannot be promoted by natural selection. On the contrary: the violators of moral laws—killers and the promiscuous—would actually reproduce much better than their victims if those offenses were a matter of genes.

Apparently, moral behavior is not just a social or genetic phenomenon, but a distinctively moral one. The following simple example may help clarify the difference: what is wrong with bullying (or any other kind of violent behavior, such as rape)? As a biological trait, it may be very advantageous to have such a gene or allele. As a social strategy, it may be a very effective strategy of banding together against a certain individual. But as a moral issue, it is plainly wrong. Those who think our actions are determined by social backgrounds, brain chemistry, and genes may be pleased to have these explanations available as escape routes from responsibility. But they may have trouble proving their point.

Morality is not under the rule of natural selection, because the moral decisions we make are not "inborn" or "useful," and therefore cannot be subject to natural selection. We do not have a moral "nature" in the physiological or genetic sense. People who act immorally do not go against their "nature"; and they are not immoral by "nature" as dictated by genes. Social behavior may very well have a genetic component, but moral behavior cannot possibly be under genetic control. A gene cannot make something obligated—perhaps more or less effective, more or less successful, but never more or less obligated. There are no genes for moral duties or moral rights.

So that leads us to the question: where do rationality and morality ultimately come from if they do not come from our genes? At this point, science has reached its limitations and boundaries; but that does not mean there is nothing beyond those boundaries. Fortunately, there is more to life than science. We can see with our "mental eyes" what no physical eyes could ever capture. It is with these mental eyes that we can discern a new dimension or perspective which opens for us a religious window on life. It is through this perspective that the only real foundation for rationality and morality can be found—in a Creator God, that is. How can that be?

If God is indeed omnipresent, "every-where," God may seem to be "no-where." So God's omnipresence only makes for God's apparent absence. Absence of evidence is not evidence of absence. As the saying goes, the last thing a fish would ever discover is water. Something similar holds for God's existence. God is also called the Primary Cause, who cannot be found among the secondary causes he created in this universe—God is not one of them. God is the First Cause—a cause that has no cause—and it is precisely for that reason he is called *first*.

Yet we have some very powerful indications of God's existence. Just think of the following series of (rhetorical) questions: How could nature be intelligible if it were not created by an intelligent Creator? How could there be order in this world if there were no orderly Creator? How could there be scientific laws if there were no rational Lawgiver? How could there be design in nature, if there were no intelligent Designer? How could there be moral laws, if there were no moral Lawgiver? How could there be human minds, if the universe were mindless? How could there be human freedom if there were no God who has freely created us after his own image?

The answer to all of these questions can only go in two directions: either there is no explanation, or there is only one explanation, God. Choosing to answer that there is no explanation is basically an irrational response that leaves us stuck in a purely material universe. Take the law of gravity—it may help us explain other things, but it cannot explain itself. Those who embrace materialism cannot dodge the question of how matter can ever explain itself, its own existence. Matter cannot just pop up out of nothing—nothing comes from nothing, as the saying goes. A solely material universe is essentially an absurd, irrational, and inexplicable universe—which is a stance that defies rationality. It must be admitted, though, that there is simply no rational way of changing the minds of people who reject rationality.

Therefore, there seems to be a compelling reason to opt for the only *rational* alternative: only the existence of God can explain that there is a universe, that there is order in this universe, that this universe is intelligible, that there are laws of nature, and that there are moral laws. This is the only way we can take the world as something created according to an intelligible plan accessible to the human intellect through the natural light of reason. Because there is a Creator, we have not only a rational Lawgiver—who guarantees order, intelligibility, and predictability—but also a moral Lawgiver—who guarantees decency, integrity, responsibility, justice, and human dignity backed by human rights. This fact led Benedict XVI to rephrase the famous philosophical rule stating that "*ought* does not flow from *is*" into its opposite as seen from a religious perspective: "The *ought* does flow from the *is*." What he meant is that once we get a sense of who God *is* and who God has destined us to *be*, certain "oughts" do become apparent. Seen in that light, our universe has been outfitted with a (moral) natural law as well as with (scientific) laws of nature. As Albert Einstein once put it, "Everyone who is seriously involved in the pursuit of science becomes convinced that a Spirit is manifest in the laws of the universe." If we do not accept this answer, then we have effectively given up on rationality and morality, for they would then be utterly baseless.

Needless to say, rationality and morality are closely intertwined. Rationality gives us reason to *defend* what is morally right; it also give us reason to *reject* what is morally wrong. And morality gives us the *duty* to pursue what is rationally true; it also gives us the *right* to defend what is rationally true. Because of this interaction, a flawed rationality always has an impact on morality, and a defective morality likewise affects rationality. In other words, rationality and morality were given to us not as qualifications we already possess but rather as capacities that we can and should use. If you ever wonder why there is so much irrationality and immorality in this world, think of this: Rationality and morality are not inborn, so they have to be taught, chosen, cultivated, and nurtured—otherwise, they wither. According to an old tale, each person harbors a good animal as well as a bad animal inside. One of the two will win, depending on which one you feed.

We could also explain this in terms of maturity. Usually grown-ups are more mature than youngsters, but we should not be surprised when a ten-year-old shows more maturity then a fifty-year-old who never matured due to lack of spiritual "nourishment." If you think you have gained maturity "through your genes," be aware that parents and children not only share their genes but also their environment, and that this holds for children even as early as in the womb. Of course children do learn from their parents, and later on from their peers as well. On the one hand, a good role model can be very contagious; on the other hand, one rotten apple can spoil the whole barrel. But in any case, all of these considerations assume one further tenet: the existence of freedom of will.

Freedom and Free Will

If everything is ruled and determined by physical, chemical, and biological laws—as some of the previous chapters seemed to suggest, to at least a certain degree—would there still be room left for our free will? The freedom of will has at least two dimensions: there is freedom as a (rational) capacity, and then there is freedom as a (moral) right. Just as words like *human* and *normal* have a descriptive sense as well as a prescriptive sense, so does the word *freedom*—it describes the way things *are*, yet it prescribes the way things *ought* to be. Let us keep that distinction in mind and begin by considering freedom as a capacity.

Having a free will is essential for us to be masters rather than victims of our actions. Free will is a rational and moral capacity that allows us to make our own choices and decisions on our life's journey. It is thanks to this free will that we can and do shape our own lives. Human freedom means that one is able to make decisions and act according to the "dictates" of one's own will—which is the freedom of self-determination. But the pivotal question is this: do we really have such freedom, or is that idea just an illusion? One thing is clear: if everything in this world were fully in the iron grip of scientific laws, including the laws of genetics, we would only be marionettes in a world of "law and order"—a viewpoint that is usually called determinism.

If determinism were an all-pervading, inescapable phenomenon in this world, such a view would certainly create trouble for all those who claim that humans have a free will. And yet, having a free will is essential for us to be masters of our actions, not victims. So do we really have a free will as a rational capacity? The facts seem to speak for themselves. Unlike animals, human beings have a strong desire to become someone of their own making. Admittedly, animals may have drives, impulses, instincts, and motives, but these are very different from intentions or reasons; not only are they mostly inborn, they also are always directly or indirectly related to sex or food. Even when it comes to food, humans often prefer to cook it before eating it—an idea that animals have never come up with.

Besides, humans have the power of reason to guide them when emotions threaten to take over. In addition, we have many other kinds of goals in life; to paraphrase the song from *South Pacific*, if you do not have a goal, how are you going to make a goal come true? Not only do humans live their lives under the influence of role models, they also steer their lives guided by reasons, purposes, plans, beliefs, values, hopes, dreams, and ideals. How different this is in the animal world—in the course of its life, an animal does not change much; it just looks and acts older and more worn-out. Humans, on the other hand, may have gone through dramatic changes in outlook on life, attitude, career, wisdom, faith, and beliefs—and all this hopefully for the better. The doctrine of complete determinism would not allow for such free decisions and choices, because everything in life is supposedly fully predetermined and preordained. However, there are some serious questions regarding this view. Is determinism truly an all-pervasive phenomenon? Is our universe really entirely at the mercy of "law and order"? Is everything in this world truly under the strict control of predetermined chains of causes and effects? Does the rigid "law-and-order" world that we live in and that science tells us about really nullify one of the privileges we thought we had, human freedom—the rational capacity to choose freely?

What reasons could we give to defend our capacity to choose freely? First of all, determinism in its all-pervasive form is self-defeating—if we consider it true, then it becomes false. When I say that all human beings are liars, then the very statement I am making as a human being must be a lie too. Similarly, when determinism wants to include everything in the universe, it must include the doctrine of determinism as well. Believing in complete determinism takes us into a vicious circle: If there is only room for predetermined things in determinism, then the claim of determinism must be one of those predetermined things—so it is not something I can freely claim, let alone deny. The doctrine of "hard" determinism creates contradictions and ultimately destroys itself; to maintain it would no longer be a reasonable belief but a physical necessity. If I am certain that everything is predetermined, I would have no reason to suppose that this certainty qualifies as true or false—and hence I would have no reason to be certain that everything is predetermined.

Second, determinism may apply within very specific and restricted scientific settings, but it cannot just be transferred to what is outside those settings. The following example may explain this. When we watch a game on the golf course or on the pool table, we see balls following precisely determined courses of cause and effect; they follow physical laws and are subject to well-known constraints; they can be explained with models that physics offers us. But there is one element that does not seem to fit in this pre-determined picture, in this cascade of causes and effects—the players of the game themselves. They may work with a physical model in their minds but they themselves are not part of that model. That is why the direction of something like a billiard ball on the pool table, or a golf ball on the golf course, is not only ruled by physical laws but also by human intentions—by players who have a certain goal in mind. And those very intentions do have consequences; they can become causes that are not part of the physical model but may still have physical or non-physical effects of their own. In the midst of physical causes, the mind can create non-physical causes of its own.

Although, in this example, we have a cascade of physical causes and effects, there is actually much more going on—these players have a very specific intention in mind, which eludes and transcends the laws of science. Do these players go *against* the laws of nature? Of course, they do not; but they do go *beyond* those laws. People who cannot look beyond those physical laws and causes are completely missing out on what the game is all about. These players somehow fall outside the realm of the model of physics, as they themselves can steer the course of the laws of nature.

In other words, even in a world ruled by the law of cause-and-effect, there is also our own ability—at a "higher" level, so to speak—to be the cause of events all by ourselves; but that ability exists beyond the physical model, invisible to the physical eye. Although chains of cause and effect appear to be very fixed and rigid, they can obviously be used and channeled within more extensive settings or designs. Think of cardiopulmonary resuscitation (CPR), for instance: applying chest compressions after cardiac arrest is not going against laws of nature, but it does go beyond the laws of nature. It uses knowledge of the laws of nature to stop the cardiac arrest.

One word of caution. Freedom of self-determination does not mean, of course, that we can do whatever we choose! When calling this universe orderly, we mean that it is law-abiding—but not necessarily pre-ordained in an iron grip. So the freedom of self-determination does not let us do whatever we want to do, but rather leaves us a series of options, curbed by a set of lawful constraints such as those known from physics, biology, psychology, sociology, economics, or history. The more we are aware of these constraints, the more we can actually be free. An ancient inscription at Delphi reads, "Know Yourself." With the proper knowledge, we can take charge of our constraints so that we are no longer their victims, but rather their architects.

When we say, for instance, that people deserve praise for their inventions, that they should be criticized for their wrong ideas, that they are held justly responsible for a crime, or that they deserve a reward for a heroic act of self-sacrifice, we mean, in the words of the British philosopher David Large, that they were the authors and causes of what they did in such a fashion that they had it in their power *not* to do what they did. Human freedom (as a capacity) is the basis of praise and blame, merit and reproach. It seems that human beings can be causes on their own, apart from any physical causes around them. On the other hand, because we have the capacity of making our own choices, we also have the freedom to be rationally wrong and morally wrong. We certainly can make mistakes, even willingly. That is the inevitable flip-side.

Apart from human freedom as a rational *capacity*, there is also human freedom as a moral *right*. Not only do we have the capacity to make choices in life, but we also have the duty and the right to make our own choices in life. Others have the duty to respect my moral rights, including my human freedom; and I have the right to expect them to respect my freedom. So the question is where this right of human freedom comes from. It certainly does not come from the government. The government can hand out entitlements, but not rights; the government cannot give rights away, although it may sometimes try to take them away.

Where do these moral rights come from, then? We discussed earlier that morality does not come from the animal world and is not etched in our genes. Yet morality tells us what we ought to do to others and what others ought to do to us; it gives us moral rights and moral duties; it gives us moral responsibilities that reinforce what "by nature" we would not desire to do anyway. What is it, then, that makes morality such a demanding issue—one indeed claiming absolute authority—if it is only a matter of genes, or tradition, or majority rule, or political correctness? Do my genes, or any other natural factors, have the right to demand absolute obedience from a person? Would society have the right to demand our absolute obedience? Would any individual have the right to demand my absolute obedience? None of the above!

The only authority that can obligate us is something—or rather Someone—infinitely superior to any of us; no one else has the right to demand our absolute obedience in matters of human dignity, human freedom, and the like. Moral rights and duties are absolute, objective standards of human behavior—they are nonnegotiable. We are responsible for the moral choices we make in life. Yes, we do have a choice when it comes to morality; but that does not mean we can choose whatever we want. We cannot just vote to decide whether we are anti-slavery and anti-abortion. Abraham Lincoln put it well when he challenged the Nebraska bill of 1820 that allowed residents to vote to decide if slavery would be legal in their territory: "God did not place good and evil before man, telling him to make his choice." There is no "pro-choice" in morality. In other words, we are under a higher Authority, in spite of the fact that many claim nowadays that there is no higher authority than "Me, Myself, and I."

Even the U.S. Declaration of Independence acknowledged that rights do not come from humans and their government, but from God. They are not man-made but God-given: "We hold these truths to be self-evident, that all men are created equal, that they are endowed by their Creator with certain unalienable Rights, that among these are Life, Liberty and the pursuit of Happiness." When in 1948 the United Nations (UN) affirmed in the *Universal Declaration of Human Rights* that "all human beings are born free and equal in dignity and rights," it must have assumed the same—otherwise all those rights would be sitting on quicksand, subject to the mercy of lawmakers and majority votes. To put it differently, human rights are not *man*-made entitlements but *God*-given rights that we cannot invent or manipulate at will.

Even an atheist like the late French philosopher Jean-Paul Sartre realized that there can be no absolute and objective standards of right and wrong if there is no eternal Heaven that would make moral values objective and universal. As he put it in his atheistic terms, it is "extremely embarrassing that God does not exist, for there disappears with Him all possibility of finding values in an intelligible heaven. There can no longer be any good a priori, since there is no infinite and perfect consciousness to think it." The German philosopher Friedrich Nietzsche was another atheist who also understood how devastating the decline of religion is for the morality of society, writing, "God is dead: but as the human race is constituted, there will perhaps be caves for millenniums yet, in which people will show his shadow.... All of us are his murderers." Nietzsche is saying here that humanism and other "moral" ideologies shelter themselves in caves and venerate shadows of the God they once believed in; they are holding on to something they cannot provide themselves, mere shadows of the past. They are "idols" constructed to preserve the essence of morality—but without the substance. This view makes it very clear that there cannot be any morality without God, for such a morality would be baseless.

Indeed, in a world without divine and eternal laws neither our human dignity nor our human freedom would be able to survive. Even the non-religious philosopher Jürgen Habermas expressed his conviction that the ideas of freedom and social co-existence are based on the Jewish notion of justice and the Christian ethics of love: "Up to this very day there is no alternative to it."

All these considerations indicate that morality comes from Heaven. We ought to do what we ought to do—for Heaven's sake! In response to Immanuel Kant, who said we should all start acting in a way that is moral "even if God does not exist," one could argue that we should do the opposite and live a moral life "as if God existed." Is it not true that, without God, we could not claim any of those rights we think we have the right to claim? Without God, we would have no (moral) rights, but only (legal) entitlements, which can be taken away at any time. President John F. Kennedy put it well in his Inaugural Address: "the rights of man come not from the generosity of the state, but from the hand of God."

So we must come to the conclusion that human freedom still stands tall: we can only be rational and moral beings because we were created with a free will—the capacity and the right to choose are always ours. We have the freedom to accept or reject what is true and what is false—as we see happening all the time—because truth and falsehood are not written in our genes. And we have the freedom to accept or reject what is right and what is wrong—as we see happening all the time—because right and wrong are not encoded in our genes.

Without God, we would almost literally lose our mind. All that we believe to be true and all that we believe to be right can only be trusted if there is a God. Without God, even an oath becomes meaningless. We can find God in every truth we discover and every good we do. If God had not given us the gift of free will, we could not be rational and moral beings who can and ought to make rational and moral decisions. Of course, we also have the freedom to decide otherwise.

Addictions

If we do have free will, how is it possible that so many people are struggling with addictions that they seem to be unable to break? Many in our society are addicted to alcohol, to nicotine, to drugs, to overeating, to compulsive shopping, to gambling, to pornography, to excessive cell-phone use, to endless video games—the list could go on and on. Are these people morally flawed, or are they perhaps lacking in willpower? Let us try to find out.

In general, we distinguish between two kinds of addictions: substance addictions (alcohol, drugs, etc.) and behavioral addictions (gambling, sex, etc.). Nonetheless, what all addictions have in common is that they go after some form of pleasure. Pleasure is what distinguishes an addiction from obsessive-compulsive disorder. While people who have addictions suffer all kinds of discomforts, the desire to use a specific substance or engage in a specific behavior is based on the expectation that it will be pleasurable. In contrast, people who experience a compulsion as part of obsessive-compulsive disorder may not get any pleasure from the behavior they engage in. Pleasure does play an important role in our lives, no doubt. If eating food and having sex did not stimulate feelings of pleasure and reward, we would expire quickly for want of food, and we would die out for want of progeny—natural selection would take care of that! These are naturally rewarding behaviors. So in a sense, everyone has some kind of addiction. It is estimated that at least 90% of Americans have at least one form of "soft" addiction in their lives. While it is healthy to relieve stress with "enjoyable" behaviors such as drinking coffee and watching television, when these become habitual they can also be problematic for one's health and happiness.

That is where the "real" addictions come into play, although the borderlines are often fuzzy. However, in general, habits and patterns associated with addictions are usually characterized by short-term rewards—some immediate pleasure—coupled with long-term costs—some delayed damaging effects. Unfortunately, we live in a society that puts great emphasis on "cheap" pleasures and "instant" gratification—while seeking to avoid any discomforts in life. All of us live in a world that runs away from discomforts. Since the time of our youth, we have been conditioned to view them as an impediment to happiness. Even a simple headache can send us hurrying to the medicine cabinet for a speedy cure. This worldview, which is so embedded in our culture, tells us that the less distress we experience, the happier we will be.

Indeed, our brains are wired to ensure that we will repeat life-sustaining activities by associating those activities with *pleasure* or reward. It is the limbic system that contains the brain's reward circuit—it lies on both sides of the thalamus, right under the cerebrum, and it links together a number of brain structures that control and regulate our ability to feel pleasure. The limbic system is activated when we perform such activities. It has a dopamine-rich area, which is an intersection where all addictive behaviors meet. Whenever this reward circuit is activated, the brain notes that something "great" is happening that needs to be remembered, and motivates us to do it again and again, without thinking about it.

Let us discuss first the mechanism behind *substance* addiction. Reasons for taking drugs or other addictive substances are various—to feel good, to feel better, to do better, to do what others do, to find out what others feel (curiosity)—but the ultimate reward is always pleasure, at least in some form and at least in the short term. Most abusive substances directly or indirectly target the brain's reward system by flooding the circuit with dopamine. Dopamine is a neurotransmitter present in regions of the brain that regulate movement, emotion, cognition, motivation, and feelings of pleasure. Overstimulation of this system produces the euphoric effects sought by people who abuse drugs, and then stimulates them to repeat the behavior. These drugs can release from two to ten times the amount of dopamine that natural rewards do. In some cases, this occurs almost immediately (as when drugs are smoked or injected), and the effects can last much longer than those produced by natural rewards. The resulting effects on the brain's pleasure-circuit dwarf those produced by naturally rewarding behaviors such as eating a regular meal. The effect of such a powerful reward strongly motivates people to take drugs again and again.

The brain adjusts to the overwhelming surges in dopamine by producing less dopamine or by reducing the number of receptors that can receive those signals. As a result, the impact of dopamine on the reward-circuit can become abnormally low, and hence the ability to experience any pleasure is reduced. Over time, if substance abuse continues, pleasurable activities become less pleasurable, and more abuse becomes necessary for abusers to simply feel "normal." Alcohol addiction, better known as alcoholism, works similarly—although the habituation process may take a bit longer than for drug addiction. The driving force is again pleasure, at least in the short run. When we drink alcohol, most of the ethanol in the body is broken down in the liver by an enzyme called alcohol dehydrogenase (ADH), which transforms ethanol (C_2H_5OH) into a toxic, unpleasant compound called acetaldehyde (CH_3CHO), also known to be a carcinogen. However, acetaldehyde is generally short-lived; it is quickly broken down into a less toxic compound called acetate (CH_3COO^-) by another enzyme called aldehyde dehydrogenase (ALDH). Acetate is finally broken down into carbon dioxide and water, mainly in tissues other than the liver.

Regardless of how much a person consumes, the body can only metabolize a certain amount of alcohol every hour. That amount varies widely among individuals and depends on a range of factors, including liver size and body mass, but also different alleles that cause differences in ADH and ALDH enzymes. Some of these enzyme variants work either more or less efficiently than others. A fast-acting ADH enzyme or a slow-acting ALDH enzyme can cause toxic acetaldehyde to build up in the body, creating dangerous and unpleasant effects.

The type of ADH and ALDH people carry has been shown to influence how much they drink, which in turn influences their risk of developing alcoholism. For example, high levels of acetaldehyde make drinking unpleasant, resulting in facial flushing, nausea, and a rapid heartbeat—which usually takes the pleasure away. On the other hand, when individuals experience strong positive (and weak negative) effects from alcohol, due to their biochemical profile, their expectations of the positive effects from the substance can be boosted, which in turn increases their desire for continued use, often resulting in dependence.

Much of the same goes for other addictive substances such as food, nicotine, caffeine, and chocolate. When analyzing a food-addiction, for example, researchers have found that the same molecular mechanisms that steer people into drug addiction are behind the drive to overeat, pushing people into obesity. They found a particular receptor in the brain known to play an important role in vulnerability to drug addiction—dopamine receptor D2. Receptor D2 responds to dopamine, which is released in the brain by pleasurable experiences after eating certain foods.

The same holds for lighting your first cigarette: although this always makes for an unpleasant experience, this does not deter everyone from trying again. Nicotine acts on nicotinic acetylcholine receptors and increases their activity, which leads to increased levels of dopamine in the reward-circuits of the brain. Again, the immediate effect is some apparent euphoria and relaxation, thereby encouraging further use, and leads to nicotine withdrawal symptoms when it is absent. There is also a strong association between depression and smoking; a lifetime history of major depression is more than twice as common in people who smoke as in people who do not. For those with a history of major depression, smoking may be an attempt to decrease negative feelings.

It is not much different with *behavioral* addictions such as relentless gambling, porn addiction, and addiction to using the internet or cellphones or video games. There are many similarities in the neurobiology of substance and behavioral addictions. They are both dependent on reinforcement and on reward-based learning processes. Take an addiction to pornography, which may start in a rather "harmless" way but gets progressively worse. The brain seeks more vile images to produce the initial effect. Several structures of the brain are important in the conditioning process of behavioral addiction. One of the major areas of study includes the region called the amygdala, which is part of the limbic system and involves emotional significance and associated learning. Behavioral addictions trigger the dopamine reward system with the following steps: the behavior causes dopamine neurons to stimulate areas along fast transmission pathways, which intensifies the behavior; this response then stimulates the neurons to send more stimuli. Once the behavior is triggered, it is hard to counteract the dopamine reward system.

Let us go back to our original question: if we have free will, how is it possible that so many people are struggling with addictions that they seem to be unable to break? Is there a genetic cause that makes them turn to a particular addiction? It does not seem so. In spite of some claims to the contrary, there is no clear evidence that there are genes that force us to become addicted. There may be genes, for instance, that affect alcohol *metabolism*, as mentioned earlier, but that does not mean they also affect alcohol *consumption*. All they do is give certain people unpleasant experiences after only one or two drinks, which may stop them from drinking sooner than others.

In general, I would maintain, there are no genes for addictions.

Genes may regulate how we react to addictions, but it is very doubtful whether they directly cause addictions. Alcohol consumption, for instance, has increased dramatically in Western societies recently, making it highly unlikely that this is a genetic phenomenon; as to nicotine addiction, for instance, the opposite has happened due to extensive anti-smoking campaigns. No one would assume that genetic changes would occur in such a short period of time. Here we have a nature-nurture issue again. To use an analogy, it is unlikely that there is a gene for "electro-shock avoidance"; we try to avoid electro-shocks only because they are very unpleasant. Call that inborn, if you want, but that is where genetics ends.

We may conclude from this that the initial decision to engage in any kind of substance addiction or behavioral addiction is mostly *voluntary*—at least it starts that way. There may be factors, though, that veer the decision in the wrong direction—such as stress, depression, low self-esteem, or a need to fit in with a group of friends. Yet, the decision-making itself is an essential part of human freedom, called self-control. Unfortunately, if the initial decision goes the wrong way, it can have very negative long-term consequences, often ending up beyond our control.

Once substance abuse takes over, a person's ability to exert self-control can become seriously impaired. Brain-imaging studies of drug-addicted individuals show physical changes in those areas of the brain that are critical to judgment, decision-making, learning and memory, and behavior control. Scientists believe that these physical changes alter the way the brain works, and may help explain the destructive behaviors of addiction. Addicts may think they are in control, but their addiction actually has come to control them.

An added problem for the power of self-control is the fact that, at a young age, the part of the brain that coordinates self-control may not be fully developed yet (free will can only work with the tools it has at its disposal). One of the brain areas still maturing during adolescence, as we have already discussed, is the prefrontal cortex—the part of the brain that enables us to assess situations, make sound decisions, and keep our emotions and desires under control. The fact that this critical part of the brains is still a work-in-progress in adolescents puts them at a higher risk for poor decision-making (such as experimenting with drugs, and then perhaps continued abuse). One of the most important behavioral changes produced by these brain changes during adolescence is an increase in the ability to exercise control over impulsive urges—as long as it does not happen too late.

This takes us to the next question: is there still a way out once someone is caught up in the cycle of any substance or behavioral addiction? The answer is a definite "yes." Addiction need not be a life sentence. Like other chronic diseases, addiction can be managed successfully. Treatment enables addicts to counteract their addiction's powerful disruptive effects on brain and behavior in order to regain control over their lives. Research shows that combining treatment medications (where available) with behavioral therapy is the best way to ensure success for most patients.

When patients first stop abusing drugs, they can experience a variety of physical and emotional symptoms, including restlessness, sleeplessness, depression, anxiety, or other mood disorders. Certain treatment medications are designed to reduce these symptoms, which makes it easier to stop the abuse. Here are some examples of such medications: for nicotine addiction, nicotine replacement therapies, bupropion, or varenicline; for opioid addiction, methadone, buprenorphine, or naltrexone; for alcohol and drug addiction, naltrexone, disulfiram, or acamprosate.

In addition, there are behavioral treatments that help engage patients in addiction treatment, modifying those attitudes and behaviors related to substance abuse and increasing their skills in handling stressful circumstances and environmental cues that may trigger intense craving for certain substances and behaviors. Another target of treatment, which is often overlooked, is self-soothing. Addicted people often use their addictions to self-soothe in stressful situations. However, since their addictions do not actually soothe them, they feel the need to take even more of the object of their addiction. It is like drinking salt water—the more you drink of it, the thirstier you get.

As to the question of free will, we should conclude the following: we usually *start* addictions voluntarily, and we can *end* them voluntarily. Self-control, or self-mastery, is training in human freedom.

The two contrasting choices we have are clear: either we govern our passions and find peace, or we let ourselves be dominated by them and become unhappy. We need to become masters of our feelings and emotions again—which is a life-long task. Self-control is not inborn but belongs to the realm of rationality and morality. It must be taught and nurtured by ridding oneself of all slavery to unruly passions. But then again, often it is hard to do all of this all on one's own.

Therefore, getting help from others who went, or are still going, through a similar process can be vital. There are now over 200 self-help organizations with a membership of millions worldwide: Alcoholics Anonymous, Narcotics Anonymous, Cocaine Anonymous, Crystal Meth Anonymous, Pills Anonymous, Marijuana Anonymous, Gamblers Anonymous, Overeaters Anonymous, Sexual Compulsives Anonymous, Sexaholics Anonymous, and Workaholics Anonymous.

All these organizations employ some kind of adjusted version of the *Twelve Steps* principles for recovery that were initially published by Alcoholics Anonymous (and were influenced by Fr. Edward Dowling, S.J.). Here are those Twelve Steps:

1. We admitted we were powerless over alcohol—that our lives had become unmanageable. 2. We came to believe that a Power greater than ourselves could restore us to sanity. 3. We made a decision to turn our will and our lives over to the care of God as we understood Him. 4. We made a searching and fearless moral inventory of ourselves. 5. We admitted to God, to ourselves, and to another human being the exact nature of our wrongs. 6. We were entirely ready to have God remove all these defects of character. 7. We humbly asked Him to remove our shortcomings. 8. We made a list of all persons we had harmed, and became willing to make amends to them all. 9. We made direct amends to such people wherever possible, except when to do so would injure them or others. 10. We continued to take personal inventory, and when we were wrong, promptly admitted it. 11. We sought through prayer and meditation to improve our conscious contact with God as we understood Him, praying only for knowledge of His will for us and the power to carry that out. 12. Having had a spiritual awaken-

ing as the result of these steps, we tried to carry this message to alcoholics, and to practice these principles in all our affairs.

Now is probably the right moment to give this discussion a more philosophical twist. Pleasures undoubtedly play an important role in life, but there is more to life than pleasure. We do have a natural desire for pleasures, but a natural desire need not be an unruly or disordered desire. This distinction stands in strong contrast to what some worldviews proclaim. Hedonism, for instance, is a school of thought that argues that pleasure is the only intrinsic good in life. Its slogan is, in essence, "it's all about pleasure"—the pleasure of food, drinks, drugs, sex, money, and what have you. It is one of those "isms" that narrow everything down to one aspect of life—actually one small part of the brain, the limbic system—while ignoring how much more there is to life. They seem broad-minded but are actually very narrow-minded, claiming that there is no other valid point of view. Hedonism is in fact another form of addiction.

In contrast, it could be argued that unlimited searching for pleasure only leads us into trouble. It leads to excess and makes people over-dosed, over-loaded, over-fed, or over-sexed—you name it. In short, it opens the gate for addictions. Addictions are a threat to everyone who places top priority on pleasure—pleasures for "Me, myself, and I." Instead, we need to learn how to control any desire for pleasure by keeping it within its healthy limits. We need to exert control over excess by self-discipline, which is something that has to be learned as early as possible—for it is not inborn. Perhaps it is something we had learned already as children when our parents taught us delayed gratification—rejecting an immediate, smaller award for a delayed, larger reward (see Chapter 3). Training our desires is like training our muscles—initially fatigued but stronger over time with frequent exercise.

In order to prepare ourselves for life, we need to control our appetites and emotions; for a life without challenge is a life without interest. Life is not all fun and games. The more one is prepared for that inevitable fact of life, the lower one's chances are of falling into a depression, which can easily be followed by an addiction. However, the tools of self-control and self-discipline are not rooted in our genes but in our upbringing. They have to be learned—and the sooner, the better. You have a better chance in life if your parents have already helped you and taught you to acquire these virtues. Clearly, no one likes discipline. Although it is a function of our uniquely human features of rationality and morality, discipline must battle with the pleasure-impulses of the limbic system that we share with the animal world.

The reality is that we do not live in a hedonistic paradise. As the philosopher Hugh J. McCann puts it, this world is not a place in which comfort and convenience are maximized, in which everyone has an electrode implanted to cause intense euphoria and ecstasy in the limbic system with a simple push of the button. We should ask ourselves the question: do we really admire those who appear to have a life of ease? What most of us do admire instead are lives of courage and sacrifice; we have a high regard for people who overcome hardship, deprivation, or weakness so as to achieve some notable success; people who stand against some great evil, or who relinquish their own pleasures to alleviate the sufferings of others. Apparently, the maximization of creaturely pleasure does not really seem to be a top priority in most lives. And if it does, addictions lurk on the horizon. When things get tough in life—and they always do at some point—the shortest road to addiction is to dull yourself and nurse your pleasures.

Let us conclude this section with something said earlier: freedom of self-determination does not mean that we can do whatever we wish or choose. Since freedom is not free, we have to fight for it. With the proper knowledge, we can take charge of our constraints so that we are no longer their victims, but rather their architects. We encounter here a peculiar situation: those who *believe* their addiction is a chronic and genetic phenomenon are less likely to kick the habit. Perhaps a better understanding of the basics of addiction will empower us to make better-informed choices in our own lives. As much as there are environmental factors—home, family, friends, school, work, or co-workers—that lure people into addiction, there are also environmental factors that *protect* them from such addictions.

5

Physical Decline

THE BIOLOGY BEHIND IT

What we discovered in the previous section about the way adults grow in maturity might give us the impression that "the sky is the limit." Unfortunately, most growing processes level off; they follow a so-called sigmoidal, or S-shaped, curve consisting of a slow starting phase and then a phase of rapid growth followed by a final phase of stagnation—or even decline. When it comes to human life, there seems to be an unavoidable moment when decline sets in, indeed irreversibly.

Going Downhill?

We all know the symptoms. Aging is a highly complex process characterized by functional decline, reduced reproductive capacity, and an increase in the likelihood of disease and death. Bones get more brittle, muscles get weaker, blood vessels become more clogged, and hair turns grayer and thinner.

One of the most visible signs of aging is hair loss. Although hair loss increases with age, it affects men more than women. The explanation is that hair loss is strongly affected by hormone levels, especially that of testosterone—more in specific di-hydro-testosterone (DHT), a derivative of testosterone. In addition, genes can make certain hair follicles more sensitive to this hormone (usually in the front and crown of the head). Hair loss is not as prevalent in women because women have more estrogen than men, which in turn helps balance out the "balding" effects of testosterone. Although women do not have nearly as much testosterone as men, when women undergo intense stress, the adrenal glands become overworked due to an increased production of adrenaline and testosterone in response—and hence increased hair loss may be the result, even for women. In general, baldness increases with age and affects 73.5% of men and 57% of women aged 80 and over.

Unfortunately, much more than hair loss occurs when people get older. With increasing age, sensory and perceptual functions start decreasing. The rate of decreasing sensory abilities varies from person to person. Vision problems are probably the most common experience. Age-related changes occur in the proteins inside the lens of the eye, making the lens harder and less elastic over time. Age-related changes also take place in the muscle fibers surrounding the lens. With less elasticity, the eye has a harder time focusing up-close. Like gray hair and wrinkles, age-related farsightedness (presbyopia) is a symptom caused by the natural course of aging—you cannot escape it, even if you never have had a vision problem before. By the time people reach the age of 75, reduced vision is very common; cataracts become more frequent as well. Furthermore, peripheral vision, depth perception, color vision, and adaptation to the dark also become poorer, and sensitivity to glare becomes stronger, which affects activities such as reading and driving a car at night.

In addition to vision deterioration, hearing ability also drops with increasing age. Thirty-five percent of the adult population experiences some kind of hearing problem between the ages of 75 and 85; and this rate rises to 50% for those at the age of 85 and over. Hearing loss limits adults' conversation abilities and will also affect cognitive functions because adults with a hearing problem miss pieces of words and phrases, so they may not fully understand what is being said. The use of hearing aids will often help these people, although the hearing aid may amplify the loudness of what they do not want to hear, more than that of what they do want to hear. But their brains must re-learn some or all of the sounds their ears have not been able to pick up and send along during the time of hearing loss. Fortunately, the brain is designed to be malleable even at an older age; but it may take several weeks with a hearing aid before the reprogramming begins. Learning to listen to the amplified sound of a hearing aid is like trying to understand someone speaking with an unfamiliar accent. It is again a learning process.

And then there is memory loss. Memory loss from aging can start as early as 45. First it should be noted, however, that memory loss is qualitatively different in normal aging from the kind of memory loss associated with a diagnosis of Alzheimer's disease. Each of us has misplaced keys, blanked out on an acquaintance's name, or forgotten a phone number. What declines with age is one's performance on memory tasks that rely on frontal brain regions—it takes longer to learn and recall information. We are not as quick as we used to be, so we speak of a "senior moment"—or, in the words of my wife, an "intellectual overload." There is indeed some evidence that when people age, they do process things at a slower pace; but that is mostly because they know so much and have to go through so much stacked information. So the idea of an intellectual overload is not as strange as it may sound.

In fact, we often mistake this slowing of our mental processes for real memory loss. But in most cases, if we give ourselves time, the information will come to mind. In fact it is quite normal that as time passes, our ability to accurately recall events becomes diminished—and the longer the period of time that passes between the event and the attempt to recall it, the greater the chance we are going to have some memory loss surrounding the event. Sometimes a long time-interval causes us to even forget the event completely.

It is important to make a distinction here between short-term memory, which generally has a limited capacity and duration, and long-term memory, which can store much larger quantities of information for virtually unlimited duration, sometimes a whole lifespan. For example, when given a random seven-digit number, we may remember it for only a few seconds before forgetting, which reflects that it was stored in our short-term memory. On the other hand, we can remember telephone numbers for many years through repetition; this information is said to be stored in our long-term memory. Short-term memory is supported by transient patterns of neuronal communication, dependent on regions of the frontal and parietal lobes. Long-term memories, on the other hand, are maintained by more stable and permanent changes in neural connections widely spread throughout the brain. The hippocampus is essential for the consolidation of information from short-term to long-term memory, although it does not seem to store information itself.

The hippocampus belongs to the limbic system and is closely associated with the cerebral cortex, as it is located in the medial temporal lobe, underneath the cortical surface. Without the hippocampus, new memories cannot be transferred into long-term memory, and there will be a very short attention span. Furthermore, the hippocampus may be involved in changing neural connections for a period of three months or more after the initial acquisition of information. How such memories are physically stored is far from clear, but in general it is believed that their storage is associated with changes in neuronal synapses. Perhaps those changes become more limited with aging; it could also be that the hippocampus becomes less capable of coordinating these processes.

However, it is also important to be aware of ways that our health, environment, and lifestyle may affect memory loss in either a positive or negative way. As already discussed, the brain is capable of producing new brain cells and new synapses at any age, so significant memory loss is not an inevitable result of aging. But just as with muscle strength, you use it or lose it. Sometimes, even what looks like significant memory loss is in fact caused by treatable conditions and reversible external factors. One of these is depression, which can mimic the signs of memory loss. Another is vitamin-B12 deficiency—older people have a slower absorption rate for nutritional supplements. Thyroid problems are another possible cause; they can lead to memory problems such as forgetfulness and difficulty concentrating. Dehydration can also be a factor, particularly when taking diuretics or laxatives or when suffering from diabetes, high blood-sugar levels, or diarrhea.

And then there are medications that have memory loss as a possible side effect; examples are sleeping pills, antihistamines, medications for blood pressure and arthritis, antidepressants, anti-anxiety medications, and painkillers. Ironically, cholesterol-lowering drugs block the very cholesterol that is so important for synapse formation and therefore necessary for learning and retention. All of this suggests that one can do something about memory loss so to avoid being completely at its mercy.

What is probably the most devastating manifestation of physical decline during aging is a more serious kind of degeneration of the nervous system as found in cases such as Parkinson's disease (PD), multiple sclerosis (MS), and Alzheimer's disease (AD). These are diseases in which nerve cells degenerate or die—usually at a rather slow pace, taking perhaps months or years. Depending on the area of the brain or spinal cord in which the degeneration of the nerve cells occurs, the symptoms differ widely. But no matter where and when it happens, the results are distressing and sometimes even tragic. Let us discuss them in some more detail.

Parkinson's disease is caused by a gradual deterioration in certain nerve centers inside the brain—mainly in the specific centers that control movement, particularly semi-automatic movements such as swinging one's arms while walking. Deterioration of these nerve centers upsets the delicate balance between the chemicals dopamine and acetylcholine, which are essential for controlling the transmission of nerve impulses.

Multiple sclerosis can affect any part of the brain or spinal cord containing myelin-covered nerves. Again, cholesterol-lowering drugs have an adverse effect on those suffering from this disease, as myelin has an important cholesterol component. The myelin sheath feeds nutrients to the nerves within it and also speeds up the passage of electrical impulses along the nerves. When the sheath becomes inflamed and swollen, one may get a sensation of tingling, numbness, or weakness that may affect only one spot, one limb, or one side of the body, depending on which sheaths are being affected. Later symptoms may become more serious. Although in two-thirds of all cases of multiple sclerosis the first attack occurs between the ages of 20 and 40, the disease virtually never begins in people over 60. So it is not really due to an aging process, but it may get worse with age for those who already have it.

Alzheimer's disease is a form of dementia that is responsible for nearly 80% of all dementia cases. It is accompanied by a progressive loss of memory and other intellectual functions, so that those affected slowly but progressively become confused, incapable of coherent conversation, unaware of their surroundings, and generally incapacitated. The underlying cause is the loss of nerve cells and the deposition in the brain of proteins called amyloids, which are insoluble protein aggregates that arise from inappropriately folded polypeptides naturally present in the body. However, in those over 65, the early symptoms of forgetfulness may not always indicate an onset of Alzheimer disease, as many other causes may have similar effects; in these non-Alzheimer's cases symptoms will lessen when the condition in question is properly treated. In fact, some 80% of people over the age of 80 still retain normal brain function.

While research shows that up to 50% of those over age 50 experience mild forgetfulness linked to age-associated memory impairment, there is the possibility that more serious threats to memory are developing. Alzheimer's disease is certainly one such threat. This disease goes beyond mere memory loss. It is about forgetting an experience, instead of just forgetting parts of an experience. It is about forgetting how to drive a car, instead of forgetting where you parked your car. It is about forgetting recent events, instead of forgetting events from the distant past. It is about forgetting ever having known a particular person, instead of forgetting a person's name and remembering it later. In general one could say that if you are worried about your memory, it is probably not that serious; but if your relatives and friends are worried about it, then it probably is a matter of greater concern.

As an added note, do not confuse the degenerative diseases described above with mental disorders such as depression, schizophrenia, bipolar disorder (formerly called manic-depression), compulsions and obsessions, personality disorders, or psychosis. These are not caused by physical decline related to aging. And it should also be emphasized that the symptoms mentioned above as a result of certain degenerative diseases can be caused by many other factors. So do not diagnose yourself.

Programmed Cell Death

What are the causes behind these declines that come with aging? Some people think that bodies wear out the way machines do—a sort of "wear and tear" brought on by extensive long-time use. Others think that everything in nature inclines from order to disorder within isolated systems, following the second law of thermodynamics which states that the entropy of an isolated system will always increase. However, it is a defining feature of life that it is *not* an isolated system: it takes in free energy from the environment and then unloads its entropy as waste. So there must be more going on with aging than just wearing out. What could it be?

The answer is a heavy-sounding concept: programmed cell death, also called *apoptosis*. Apoptosis is a programmed form of cell death, to be distinguished from necrosis, which is an accidental form of cell death caused by disease or injury. Cells can die in two different ways: either they are killed by harmful agents or they are induced to commit "suicide." The latter—programmed cell death—is a very common phenomenon in the human body at all ages. Every day, some 500 billion blood cells are eliminated by programmed cell death in order to offset their continual production in the bone-marrow. We had seen something similar already when we discussed how neurons are produced in excess, with up to 50% subsequently eliminated by programmed cell death (see Chapter 3). Most tissues actually contain so-called stem cells which are able to replace cells that have been lost—either by accident, or by programmed cell death.

To put it in a catchphrase, for every cell there is a time to live and a time to die. In adult organisms, cell death must be balanced by cell renewal. Apoptosis plays a crucial role in developing and maintaining the health of the body by eliminating old, unnecessary, and damaged cells. The human body replaces perhaps one million cells per second. However, either too little or too much apoptosis can lead to various diseases. When apoptosis does not work often enough, cells that should be eliminated may persist and become "immortal"—for example, in cancer and leukemia. On the other hand, when apoptosis works overly well, it kills too many cells and inflicts critical tissue damage.

As mentioned already, apoptosis can be a very beneficial process. For an average child between the ages of 8 and 14, approximately 20 billion to 30 billion cells die each day due to apoptosis, and between 50 and 70 billion cells per day in adults. Apoptosis is also responsible for more specific functions. Here are some examples: the formation of the fingers and toes of the fetus requires the removal, by apoptosis, of the tissue between them; the sloughing-off of the inner lining of the uterus at the start of menstruation occurs by apoptosis; the formation of synapses, the proper connections between neurons in the brain, requires that surplus cells be eliminated by apoptosis; and the elimination of T-cells, or T-lymphocytes, that might otherwise mount an autoimmune attack on the body occurs by apoptosis.

But apoptosis can also run out of hand when it causes cell loss without replacement—which is a major cause of aging in humans. In aging organisms, cell death outpaces cell renewal. So what is it, then, that regulates apoptosis?

Apoptosis is a multi-step, multi-pathway cell-death program that is inherent in every cell of the body. It is sensitive to a diverse range of cell signals, including toxins, hormones, growth factors, or nitric oxide (NO). These signals may either induce or repress apoptosis. Repressed apoptosis can result in a number of cancers, autoimmune diseases, inflammatory diseases, and viral infections. It was originally believed that the associated accumulation of cells was due to an increase in cellular proliferation, but it is now known that it is also due to a decrease in cell death.

Some viruses (such as Epstein-Barr virus and human papilloma viruses) and some cancer cells (melanomas and some B-cell leukemias and lymphomas) use "tricks" to avoid apoptosis of the infected cells. Consequently, cancer treatment by chemotherapy and irradiation does the opposite; it kills target cells primarily by inducing apoptosis (see Chapter 6). Once we know more about the details of this mechanism, we may find better ways to induce the death of cancer cells.

To summarize: an unbalanced and overly active apoptosis is the main cause of aging; it affects almost every organ, but most noticeably the brain. Ultimately, it will most likely lead to the final stage of life's journey, which we will discuss in the last section.

BEHIND THE BIOLOGICAL FACTS

The previous section had a rather bleak ending, especially regarding brain functions. That may not be fair and balanced, however, because there is a problem with the prevailing paradigm of neuroscience. Let us take a look at what that is.

The term "paradigm," the use of which in a scientific context Thomas Kuhn introduced, indicates a collection of rules for how to solve scientific puzzles. The current paradigm of neuroscience is too materialistic and too deterministic to do justice to the unique position of human beings in this world, thus, it could be argued that it must be replaced with a new one. It is not fair to suggest that all neuroscientists nowadays adhere rigidly to the traditional paradigm, but a majority obviously does.

There is a great deal of resistance to a new paradigm, because the existing paradigm has been so successful in solving scientific problems. Scientists also tend to feel attached to the paradigm they were brought up with. Individual scientists acquire knowledge of a paradigm through their scientific education and training. That is how they learn their standards: by solving "standard" problems, performing "standard" experiments, and eventually doing research under a supervisor already skilled within the paradigm. Aspiring scientists become gradually acquainted with the methods, the techniques, and the presuppositions of that particular paradigm. Because of their training, scientists are typically unable to articulate the precise nature of the paradigm in which they work until the need arises to become aware of the general laws, metaphysical assumptions, and methodological principles involved in the paradigm. Perhaps such an awareness is what neuroscientists need in order to see the limitations of their paradigm.

The Mind Behind the Brain

Neuroscientists of the "old school"—from the old paradigm, if you will—focus exclusively on the brain, while ignoring the possibility that the *brain* may not be the same as the *mind*. In their opinion, mind-science is "nothing but" brain-science. So when the brain declines—biologically, that is—then the mind must be in decline as a consequence, so they believe. Behind this view is the assumption that the brain is the only reality, and the "mind" is something like an illusion. One could certainly challenge this assumption by claiming that the mind is different from the brain. There are many reasons for making a meaningful distinction between the two. Here are just a few.

First of all, mental activities of the mind are very different from neural activities of the brain. The German philosopher Gottfried Leibniz once suggested that we picture the brain as so greatly enlarged that one could walk in it as if in a mill. Inside, one would observe movements of several parts, but never anything like a thought. For this reason, he concluded that thoughts must be different from physical and material movements and parts. Nowadays, the mechanical model of cogs and wheels that Leibniz used has been replaced by the chemical model of biochemical pathways, but the outcome is the same. If Leibniz is right, that would explain why brain-scans never reveal thoughts; all they can pick up are "brain waves," since thoughts fail to show up on pictures and scans.

Because of this difference, we should refine our terminology: neuro-scientists are not mind-readers, neuro-surgeons are not mind-surgeons, and neuro-science is not mind-science. Simply put, thoughts are more than brain waves—in the same way as love is more than a chemical reaction. Medical professionals can read and interpret an electroencephalogram (EEG) or a magnetic resonance image (MRI), but looking at these does not show them any thoughts—perhaps memory "traces" of thoughts, but not the thoughts themselves. They simply cannot "read" your mind. All they can study is a "mind-less" brain.

Second, thoughts are immaterial and can be true or false. Whereas the brain as a material entity has characteristics such as length, width, height, and weight, the mind does not have any of these; thoughts are true or false, right or wrong, but never tall or short, heavy or light (unless taken in a figurative sense). The late Nobel Laureate Sir John Eccles stressed the difference thusly: "The more we discover about the brain, the more clearly do we distinguish between the brain events and the mental phenomena, and the more wonderful do both the brain events and the mental phenomena become."

Third, if the mind were just the brain, its thoughts would be as fragile as the molecules they supposedly came from. In contrast, we must stress that mental activities are very different from neural activities—we cannot just deny the mental, because denying the existence of mental activities is in itself a mental activity, and thus would lead to contradiction. J.B.S. Haldane argued this along the following lines: if mental processes are nothing but the motions of atoms in the brain, we have no reason to suppose that our beliefs are true… and hence we have no reason for supposing our minds to be composed of atoms. This is a profound philosophical statement that deserves serious attention; it may shake the atoms in your head.

Fourth, the brain is only the physical carrier of immaterial thoughts in the mind (see Chapter 3). Once we realize that the same thought can be transported by different vehicles—such as pen strokes on paper, currents in computers, or impulses in the brain—we must acknowledge that a thought is distinct from its carrier. If you were to break your radio, the news report would stop, but this does not mean the news was created by the radio; it was only the news vehicle that broke down. So it seems evident that the brain does not create thoughts but merely transports them. The thoughts somehow "use" the vehicle. The brain is a vehicle of thoughts coming from the mind in the same sense as a book or a CD can be a vehicle of thoughts created by someone's mind.

Fifth, consider for a moment how a neuroscientist can study the brain. The obvious question would be: could the brain ever study the brain all by itself? That would be like the magic of a projector projecting itself or a copy machine copying itself. That which studies the brain must be "more" than the brain itself—in the same way as Watson and Crick must have been "more" than the DNA they discovered and studied. We just cannot pull ourselves up by our own bootstraps. To put it in more philosophical terms, the *knowing subject* must be "more" than the *known object*.

Arguably, only the mind as a knowing subject is able to study the brain as a known object, because it requires a mind to understand the brain, just as it requires a subject to study any object. When science studies the brain, such can only be done thanks to the mind of a subject, the scientist. When studying the human brain as an object of science, a scientist needs the human mind as the subject of science—for without the human mind, with its intellect and rationality, there would be no science at all. To sum up, one would need a mind before one could study the brain. However, the mind can never really understand itself, as little as the eye can see itself or a finger can point at itself.

Sixth, it is the mind—this mysterious intellectual part of the soul—that allows us to be rational and moral beings, which fact separates us from the animal world (see Chapter 4). Since animals do not have a mind, they cannot study the brain. Humans, on the other hand, can. And they have been doing so since prehistoric times; the opening of the skull—trepanation—was already taking place during the Stone Age, without anesthesia or antisepsis. For centuries, the human mind has been studying the brain.

If our rationality and morality were merely a matter of the brain, we would have no way to distinguish between true and false, or between right and wrong. If the mental were the same as the neural, thoughts could never be right or wrong and true or false; neural events simply happen, and that is that! In addition to the five senses of sight, hearing, taste, smell, and touch that give us access to a world of material things, we have two more "senses" that give us access to what is immaterial—a world of what is true or false in a rational sense and what is right or wrong in a moral sense. Thanks to the mind, we have a rational sense of true and false as well as a moral sense of right and wrong.

Seventh, even the fact that certain mental phenomena seem to be associated with certain neural phenomena does not entail that these mental phenomena are *caused* by neural phenomena. Correlation does not imply causation. Take functional magnetic resonance imaging (fMRI), for example—an MRI procedure that measures brain activity by detecting associated changes in blood flow. When regions light up on an fMRI, that fact does not explain whether this lit-up state is causing a certain mental state or just reflecting it. It could just as well be claimed that it is the mind that makes those areas light up. Whereas something like pain can be induced in a physical way, there is no evidence that experimental stimulation of specific neuronal areas would produce a specific mental state or a specific thought.

Saying that thoughts cannot be physically induced does not hold for something like emotions or feelings (which even animals experience), because those are physical and biological phenomena that can be physically induced by stimulation of certain areas of the brain. The same can be said about memories stored in the brain—

including memories of thoughts once produced by the mind—because memories can be physically stored, similar to the way thoughts can be "stored" on paper. Thoughts, on the other hand, cannot be produced in a physical manner, let alone by electrodes. Perhaps you wish that the thought of "two times two" would physically produce the thought of "four," for you could thereby have easily skipped much time in school—but the reality is otherwise.

Eighth, neural activity not only fails to be a sufficient condition for mental activity but may not even be a necessary condition. Put differently, there may be mental activity even when there is little or no neural activity. We know of situations where the most intense subjective experiences correlate with a dampening—or even cessation—of brain activity. In particular, there can be a high level of mental activity without a corresponding high level of neural activity. What comes to mind are cases of near-death experiences (NDEs) or out-of-body experiences (OBEs) induced by G-LOC, cortical deactivation through the use of high-power magnetic fields, mystical experiences induced through hyper-ventilation, and brain damage caused by surgery or strokes (see also Chapter 6).

For all of the above reasons, body and mind seem to represent two very different aspects of the same human being; you can *tell* them apart but you cannot *set* them apart. The body and its brain belong to the world of objects, whereas mind and soul are part of the world of subjects—the mind being the intellectual part of the soul. These are two different aspects of the same human being—two aspects that we can distinguish but not separate. And yet they are both real; there is a mental aspect of reality and there is a physical aspect of reality. The fact that we can distinguish them does not entail that we can separate them, any more than the idea of a three-dimensional space means that we can actually separate those three dimensions. As to *how* body and mind interact, we do not really know.

This last statement is not as strange as it may sound. Think of the relationship between mass and gravity; we do not really know how these two interact. Or take the case of electrically charged particles that interact with each other through the mediation of electromagnetic fields; the charged particles affect the fields and the fields affect the particles, but we do not know anything about the "mechanism" behind this interaction. Something similar is the case when it comes to body and mind; we know *that* they interact but do not know *how*.

On one occasion, the late neurosurgeon Wilder Penfield asked one of his patients to try to prevent the movement of the latter's left arm, which the former was about to make move by stimulating the motor cortex in the right hemisphere of the brain. The patient grabbed his left arm with his right hand, attempting to restrict the movement that was to be induced by a surgical stimulation of the right brain. As Penfield said, "Behind the brain action of one hemisphere was the patient's mind. Behind the action of the other hemisphere was the electrode." That is the enigma of the mind in a nutshell. The mind—that "spooky" metaphysical concept, according to some—could very well be a powerful metaphysical force in a physical body.

St. Thomas Aquinas in particular has helped to place this discussion in a wider philosophical, metaphysical framework. For Aquinas, the soul is the substantial *form* of a human being. Body and soul, or spirit and flesh, are two sides of the same coin, then, as form and matter are both necessary for any material object; indeed, the soul is the form of the body, or, put differently, the spirit is the form of the flesh. Applied to the relationship between brain and mind—with the mind being the intellectual part of the soul—this would entail that the "form" of the mind gives a specific existence to the "matter" of the brain. Aquinas truly embraces the total reality of the human person as an organic composite of spirit and matter without overemphasizing one element to the detriment of the other. So there is a very tight connection between the two, as common experience testifies: an intoxicated body affects the mind, and a confused mind affects the body; stress affects the brain, and headaches affect the mind; people with an optimistic outlook on life tend to be healthier and live longer than those with a negative outlook.

Examples like these show that the unity between body and soul, or between brain and mind, is so strong that we can even speak of psycho-somatic disorders that affect the two together. However, in spite of this unity, the distinction between body and soul, between brain and mind, or between matter and form remains pivotal. The fact that an intoxicated brain cannot think well does not necessarily mean that the thinking comes from the brain. It could very well be argued that it is the mind that thinks, but it uses the brain to do so. To use the analogy of a poster: the message can be found in the "form" of the poster, but the paper of the poster is just the "matter" that carries the message.

Back to the brain. In the past sections, we talked quite a bit about the plasticity of the brain. Does that not mean that we are still at the mercy of the brain—and indirectly that of the genes behind it? Let me make clear that the plasticity of the brain is more like a passive response to new experiences than an active agent in search of new experiences. Searching for new experiences requires the creativity of the *mind*. Brain plasticity may help us cope with new experiences, but it does not create new experiences. Plasticity of the brain does not create creativity; it merely enables it. Instead of saying that creativity of the mind is a "side-effect" of the plasticity of the brain, we should rather change the roles and claim that the mind is the steering-power behind the plasticity of the brain. It is mental creativity that is capable of manipulating neural plasticity by rewiring the brain—even at an older age. Unfortunately, many severely wounded older people have had to go through intense therapy to rewire their nervous system. Brain plasticity may allow for it, but the mind needs to activate it.

Defective Brains

How does all of this relate to the stage of physical decline in the body? Regardless of what mainstream neuroscientists may decree, one could argue that physical decline in the *brain* does not necessarily mean a mental or spiritual decline of the *mind* as well. The interesting part is that it is the mind that can make the brain exercise—if it does not, it must have its reason not to do so. The mind is in charge of the brain, in spite of the fact that owing to certain biological defects the brain may not always cooperate. We all know, for instance, that the mind cannot work through an intoxicated brain, in the same way as the news cannot come in through a broken radio or TV.

In other words, one should not confuse a "defective brain" with a "broken mind." A broken brain is as physical a phenomenon as a broken bone—but the mind is not physical, nor is the soul. To be sure, thinking presupposes a functioning brain, but it cannot be reduced to this fist-sized organ. Even people who have "lost their mind"—whether it is through dementia, Alzheimer's disease, autism, or mental insanity—have not really lost their minds or their souls. What they did lose is essentially part of their brains, not their minds. The fact that they are human means that they have a human mind and a human soul. Even if their brains show fewer neural activities, or even hardly any at all, this fact does not necessarily mean that their mental activities have come to a halt as well. Defects in the physical network of neurons or neurotransmitters can prevent the mind from working through bodily activities in the way it used to—it is like the static noise in a news broadcast. If such patients did not have a mind, they would indeed merely be broken-down machines that could be discarded at any time.

Yet isn't this mere philosophical speculation? Interestingly enough, researchers at the University of Virginia and the University of Vienna, Austria are studying a phenomenon that has been called "terminal lucidity"—the unexpected return of mental clarity and memory shortly before the death of patients suffering from severe mental disorders. It is the term used when dying people, who have previously been unresponsive or minimally responsive, suddenly gain clarity of mind for a few hours, often talking coherently with loved ones before passing away a short time later. We know that there is no observable sudden change in the brain when death is very near. Is it possible, then, that the mind's sudden and short-lived return to normalcy just before death is brought about not by some inexplicable surge in brain functioning but by the mind's distancing itself from the brain? Examples of this phenomenon include case reports of patients suffering from tumors, strokes, Alzheimer's disease, and schizophrenia. Although terminal lucidity has been reported for around 250 years, it has received little scientific attention because of its complexity and transience—or perhaps because it doesn't fit into a paradigm that equates mind research with brain research.

One could argue that, in cases like Alzheimer's disease, the mind has become an "incarcerated" mind, working with the tools of a failing brain. Language skills, for example, are impacted early on in the development of Alzheimer's disease. Yet therapy may often help such people to stay in touch with their "self." In addition, encouraging the recounting of personal histories; prompting your loved one to share his or her moments of greatness; and speaking in a calm, loving, simple, yet adult manner will facilitate your interactions during the early years of the disease. In spoken communication, most of the meaning comes from tone, gestures, and other forms of body language. These nonverbal skills become all the more important as words fade. Even in the late stages of the disease, patients still communicate a great deal through eye-contact, gestures, looks, posture, nods, facial expression, and breathing patterns, and can still respond to others. Building nonverbal skills can maintain your relationship, improve your interactions, and foster a sense of well-being for you and your loved one. Or perhaps we should change the roles and say with William Shakespeare in *King Lear*, "We are not ourselves when nature, being oppressed, commands the mind to suffer with the body."

Much of the above is also true for individuals with a speech impediment, or people who are seemingly in a coma; they just cannot say verbally what they want to say. The brain hinders the mind from expressing itself. "Mind over matter" may not work at all times, since "matter" sometimes just will not cooperate with the mind. Does this mean the mind of such people is "gone"? It must be reiterated that since the mind is immaterial, we cannot record its activities—we can only do so for the brain—but those activities are still there, although more or less hidden from us in a haze.

The mind is the most personal "part" we have, allowing us to be a knowing subject of innumerable known objects. The mind is the intellectual part of the soul. Even if you had an identical twin, you would still be *you*—not him or her. You could never imagine having your mind in a different body; but when we grow older, we do learn what it feels like to have the same mind in an aging body—it can be a very humbling experience.

6

The Final Stage

THE BIOLOGY BEHIND IT

Not surprisingly, the final stage of life's journey is death. Traditionally, both the legal and medical communities defined death in terms of the end of certain bodily functions, especially respiration and heartbeat. But it is not so easy to mark the actual end of life's journey.

Clinical Death and Brain Death

"Clinical death" is the medical term for cessation of blood circulation and breathing, the two necessary conditions for sustaining biological life. It occurs when the heart stops beating in a regular rhythm, a condition called cardiac arrest. When your heart stops, your brain no longer gets the blood it needs to function, and you lose consciousness immediately—unless the heartbeat and circulation can be restored by cardiac massage within a few minutes. Prior to the invention of cardiopulmonary resuscitation (CPR), defibrillation, epinephrine injection, and other treatments in the twentieth century, the absence of blood circulation was considered to be the official definition of death.

With the advent of these new strategies, cardiac arrest came to be called *clinical death* rather than simply "death"—reflecting the possibility of post-arrest resuscitation. For medical purposes, this is considered to be the final physical state before permanent death sets in. At the onset of clinical death, consciousness is not lost until 15–20 seconds later. Measurable brain-activity stops within 20 to 40 seconds. Although most tissues and organs of the body can survive clinical death for considerable periods of time, the brain cannot. Without special treatment after circulation is restored, full recovery of the brain after more than five minutes of clinical death at normal body temperature is rare. Brain injury is therefore the limiting factor for recovery from clinical death. However, reducing body temperature by 3° Celsius after restoring blood circulation can double the time-window for recovery from clinical death without brain damage from five to ten minutes. This induced-hypothermia technique is beginning to be used in emergency medicine.

With the increasing ability of the medical community to resuscitate patients who have no respiration, heartbeat, or other external signs of life, the need for a better definition of death became obvious. This need gained greater urgency with a rising demand for organ transplantation. It is now understood that death is in fact a series of physical events, not a single one.

An ad-hoc committee at Harvard Medical School published a pivotal 1968 report defining "irreversible coma." The Harvard criteria gradually became the norm for what is now known as *brain death*. A brain-dead individual shows no clinical evidence of brain function, which entails no response to pain and no cranial nerve reflexes—no pupillary response (fixed pupils), no corneal reflexes, no oculo-vestibular reflex, no gag reflex, and no spontaneous respirations. When removed from the ventilator, the active brain will cause the patient to breathe spontaneously—due to a rise of the CO_2 level in the blood—whereas a dead brain would give no response. Although the patient has a dead brain and a dead brainstem, there may still be spinal cord reflexes that can be elicited (a knee-jerk, for example). In some brain-dead patients, when the hand or foot is touched in a particular manner the touch will still elicit a brief reflex movement.

In addition to the aforementioned clinical signs of brain death, many physicians and most state laws require additional confirmatory tests before declaring brain death. The two most common are the electroencephalogram (EEG) and the cerebral blood flow (CBF) test. The EEG measures brain voltage in microvolts. It is so sensitive that the static electricity in a person's clothes will give a squiggle on the EEG (a false positive). All real positive responses suggest brain function. The CBF test involves the injection of a mild radioactive isotope into the blood stream. By placing a radioactivity counter over the head, one can measure the amount of blood flow into the brain. If there is no blood flow to the brain during this test, the brain is considered dead. Just as one cannot be "half" pregnant, so one cannot be "half" brain-dead—brain death, like pregnancy, is either yes or no; there is no in-between.

It is important, though, to distinguish between brain death and states that may mimic brain death—such as barbiturate overdose, alcohol intoxication, sedative overdose, hypothermia, hypoglycemia, coma, or chronic vegetative states. Some comatose patients can still recover, and some patients with severe irreversible neurological dysfunction will nonetheless retain some lower brain functions such as spontaneous respiration, although both cortex and brainstem no longer function. We should mention, though, that patients who suffer brain death are not in a coma; patients in a coma may or may not progress to brain death. Then there are patients who are in what is called a "vegetative state"; they have much more lower-brain function, and a bit more upper brain-stem function, than a patient in deep coma would exhibit. In either case, though, the patient is considered legally alive, because he or she still has some neurological signs.

Why is the brain more important than the heart when it comes to death? The brain controls all our bodily functions, but there are three things it cannot do. First, it cannot feel pain; it does "receive" pain from all over the body, but not from within itself. Second, the brain cannot store oxygen, so one feels a lack of oxygen after just a few seconds. Third, the brain cannot store glucose, so it starves in a very short time. The last two conditions require a heartbeat to deliver oxygen and glucose; so when there is cardiac arrest, resuscitation has to be done within five minutes, or otherwise the body's main control-center breaks down. Although the heart can continue to beat without brain activity, all other processes in the body will gradually come to a halt when they are no longer controlled by the brain. When the brain dies, all the body's organs will inevitably collapse.

Although the electrical activity of the brain can stop completely, or drop to such a low level that it cannot be detected with most equipment, the lack of electrical activity—a flat-EEG—would not be decisive, because it sometimes also occurs during deep anesthesia or cardiac arrest. In the United States, a flat-EEG test is not required to certify death, but it is considered to have confirmatory value. Once brain death has been confirmed, we speak of "legal death," even if the heart is still beating and mechanical ventilation can keep all other vital organs completely alive and functional.

To put it bluntly, is brain-dead dead enough? The consensus is that if a person's entire brain is dead, the person is dead. The reason is that if the entire brain is destroyed, there is absence of spontaneous breathing, and cessation of heartbeat is expected to follow soon thereafter. It is on the basis of this expectation that all life-support treatments which the patient may have had in place before brain death has been confirmed can be removed on the grounds that the patient is now dead. It also provides the opportunity to obtain organs from a brain-dead patient, provided consent has been given, while the organs are still in good condition for transplantation. However, some religious groups and even some healthcare workers are uncomfortable with a brain-death definition of death, since the patient may still have a heartbeat, and so they wish to wait until there is persisting absence of heart beat—which is the classical criterion for clinical death.

Is There Endless Life?

As the saying goes, death and taxes are the two certainties in life. We could possibly abolish taxes, but could we ever abolish death? Some biologists think so. They believe there is an ultimate "cure" for human mortality.

The longest-living person whose dates of birth and death have been verified according to modern standards was Jeanne Calment, a French woman who lived to the impressive age of 122. The maximum recorded lifespan for humans has increased from 103 year in 1798 to 110 years in 1898, to 115 years in 1990, and to 122.45 years since Calment's death in 1997. Is there a way we can keep prolonging this process—perhaps even up to biological immortality?

Some believe that if we could prevent cells from aging, we could perhaps achieve biological immortality. So the question is: what makes a cell age? The indications are that *telomeres* are closely connected with cell aging. Telomeres are a region of repetitive nucleotide sequences at each end of every chromosome which protects the end of the chromosome from deterioration or from fusion with neighboring chromosomes. They resemble the plastic tips on shoelaces because they prevent chromosome ends from fraying and sticking to each other. Every time a cell divides into two new cells, the telomeres become a bit shorter. Elderly people generally have shorter telomeres than younger people. When these telomeres are finally worn down, the cell is unable to divide, and eventually dies.

However, there is an enzyme, telomerase, which rebuilds the telomeres in stem cells and cancer cells, allowing them to replicate an infinite number of times. These cells activate the DNA code for telomerase, which allows them to divide repeatedly. In adults, telomerase is highly activated in cells that need to divide regularly (e.g., stem cells and cells in the immune system), whereas most somatic cells express it only at very low levels. Interestingly enough, it has been found that negative life experiences can accelerate telomere erosion, whereas positive behaviors can stave it off. The mechanism behind this phenomenon remains puzzling.

In the laboratory, biologists have been able to culture "immortal" cell lines. The first and still most widely used immortal cell line is *HeLa*, developed from cells taken in 1951 from the malignant cervical tumor of a patient named Henrietta Lacks, albeit without her consent. These cancer cells activate the DNA code for the telomere-lengthening enzyme telomerase, and thereby avoid apoptosis (programmed cell death). As we discussed earlier, out-of-control apoptosis is the main cause of aging.

While this potential for unrestrained growth has excited many researchers, caution is warranted in manipulating this property, as this same phenomenon of unbounded growth is a crucial step in enabling cancer to develop—and we know how destructive cancer can be (see Chapter 6). There is still another reason why biological immortality is very unlikely for human beings. It has been found that the VO_2 max value (a measure of the volume of oxygen flow to the cardiac muscle) decreases with increasing age. Therefore, the maximum lifespan of an individual can be determined by calculating when his or her VO_2-max value will drop below the basal metabolic rate necessary to sustain life—which is approximately 3 ml per kg per minute.

Let us play science-fiction for a moment. Even if we would ever find a way to bring the aging process to a complete halt, we still would have to deal with traffic accidents, murders, natural catastrophes, infections, cancers—and the list could go on and on. Science may help us prevent some of these; but it is not realistic to expect miracles from science, especially not when it comes to immortality. It makes probably much more sense to take immortality off the list of attainable, let alone desirable, goals.

The Threat of Cancer

One of the most common causes of death is cancer. In total, cancers account for approximately 13% of all deaths each year. Taken as a whole, about half of those receiving treatment for invasive cancer die from cancer or its treatment, although progress is being made. No wonder cancer has a reputation as a deadly disease. However, the survival rates vary dramatically by type of cancer, with the range running from nearly all victims surviving to almost none surviving. Those who survive cancer, however, are at increased risk of developing a second primary cancer, about twice as high as with those never diagnosed with cancer. The increased risk is believed to be primarily due to the same risk factors that produced the first cancer, and partly due to the treatment for the first cancer.

Global cancer rates have been on the rise, mainly due to an aging population and lifestyle changes in the developing world. Arguably, the most significant risk factor for developing cancer is old age. Although it is possible for cancer to strike at any age, most people who are diagnosed with invasive cancer are over the age of 65. One could even say that, if we lived long enough, sooner or later we all would get cancer.

The term "cancer" covers a broad group of various diseases, all involving unregulated cell growth. Cancers are classified by the type of cell from which the tumor originated. These types of cells include carcinomas (derived from epithelial cells), sarcomas (arising from connective tissue), lymphomas and leukemias (arising from blood-forming cells), myelomas (stemming from plasma cells of bone marrow), adenomas (derived from glandular tissues), gliomas (arising from connective glial cells that support nerve cells in the brain), and germ-cell tumors in the testicles or the ovaries.

In spite of all these different varieties, cancer is fundamentally a disease of failure in regulating cell growth. Somehow a normal cell has been transformed into a cancer cell by changes in those genes which regulate cell growth and differentiation. The affected genes are divided into two broad categories. Oncogenes are genes which *promote* cell growth and reproduction. Tumor-suppressor genes are genes which *suppress* cell division and survival. Either kind can be disrupted by genetic changes called mutations.

Genetic changes can occur at the chromosome level or at the gene level. At the *chromosome* level, a portion of a chromosome containing oncogenes and/or tumor-suppressor genes can be deleted or amplified. A well-known example of this is the Philadelphia chromosome—a translocation of chromosomes 9 and 22—which occurs in chronic myelogenous leukemia, and results in production of an oncogenic enzyme called tyrosine kinase.

More common, however, are mutations at the *gene* level, effected by changing the nucleotide sequence of nuclear DNA. These mutations may occur in the promoter region of a gene and affect whether the gene comes to expression or not; or they may occur directly in the gene's coding sequence and alter the function or stability of its protein product. Disruption of a single gene may also result from integration of DNA-material that stems from a virus or retrovirus and results in the expression of viral oncogenes in the affected cell and its descendants.

How cancer sufferers end up with these mutated genes and alleles in the first place? One of the possibilities is that they inherited the mutation from their parents—which raises the question, of course, as to how their parents acquired them. However, only a small number of cancer cases are primarily caused by an inherited genetic defect—in fact, less than 3–10% of all cancers. Examples of such cases are inherited mutations in the genes BRCA1 and BRCA2, with a more than 75% risk of breast cancer, ovarian cancer, and pancreatic cancer; and mutations in the genes HNPCC, MLH1, MSH2, MSH6, PMS1, and PMS2, which can cause cancer in the colon, uterine, small intestine, stomach, and urinary tract.

Another possibility is that there are viruses involved. Viruses contain DNA or RNA; once they get incorporated into the human cell, they can interfere with cell-growth regulation. A virus that can cause cancer contains oncogenes and is called an onco-virus. Examples are the human papillomavirus for cervical carcinoma, the Epstein-Barr virus for nasopharyngeal carcinoma, the Kaposi sarcoma herpes-virus for certain lymphomas, the hepatitis-B and hepatitis-C viruses for liver carcinoma, and the Human T-cell leukemia virus-1. In addition to viral infection, bacterial infection may also increase the risk of cancer, as is seen in *Helicobacter pylori*-induced gastric carcinoma. And then there are parasitic infections that are associated with cancer.

In most cases, however, cancer is caused by environmental factors that are known as *carcinogens*. Most of these agents cause cancer by inducing harmful mutations; that is why those particular carcinogens are also called *mutagens*. One study showed that approximately 90% of all known carcinogens are mutagens. The modern environment exposes everyone to a wide variety of chemicals in drugs, cosmetics, food preservatives, food coloring, plastics, pesticides, pollutants, and so forth. Not only do they enter through the digestive tract—in which case they still pass the liver, which may destroy them—but they also enter through the skin and lungs, without having to pass the test of the liver first.

Many of these compounds have been shown to be carcinogenic as well as mutagenic. Examples include the food-preservative AF-2; the food-fumigant ethylene dibromide; the drug hycanthone; several hair-dye additives; and the industrial compound polyvinyl chloride (PVC), used in some plastics (plastic #3, used to make food wrap, bottles for cooking oil, and plumbing pipes). Acrylamides, which can be found in food that has been fried or baked at high temperatures, are also known to be carcinogenic. Recently, the National Institutes of Health (NIH) has added formaldehyde and styrene to the list of potential carcinogens; formaldehyde is used to make compounds such as plastics and synthetic fibers; styrene is a synthetic chemical used in the manufacturing of products such as rubber and plastic. The greatest exposure to styrene in the general population, however, is through cigarette-smoking.

Another infamous group of mutagens are radioactive substances such as radon; they are sometimes called radio-nuclides or radioactive isotopes. What they have in common is that they are atoms with an unstable nucleus which can cause radiation. Radiation is the release or emission of energetic particles or waves. An important distinction that affects the presence of health risk from radiation is whether the released energy is ionizing or non-ionizing.

Non-ionizing radiation is a low-frequency radiation that does not have enough energy to remove electrons or directly damage DNA. Low-energy UV-rays, visible light, infrared rays, microwaves, and radio waves are all forms of non-ionizing radiation. Aside from UV-rays, these types of radiation are not known to increase cancer risk. Ionizing radiation, on the other hand, is high-frequency radiation that has enough energy to remove an electron from an atom or molecule, thereby ionizing it. Ionizing radiation has enough energy to damage the DNA in cells, which in turn may lead to cancer. Gamma rays, X-rays, and some high-energy UV-rays are forms of ionizing radiation. The amount of damage in the cell is related to the dose of radiation it receives.

It is important to understand the difference between these two types of radiation. For example, the non-ionizing radiation given off by a cell phone or a television screen is not the same as the ionizing radiation one might get from X-rays taken in the hospital. Ionizing radiation, on the other hand, is a proven human carcinogen. The evidence for this comes from many different sources, including studies of atomic bomb survivors in Japan, people exposed during the Chernobyl nuclear accident, patients treated with high doses of radiation for cancer and other conditions, and people exposed to high levels of radiation at work, such as uranium miners, or at home (radon). In general, the risk of cancer from this kind of radiation-exposure increases as the dose of radiation increases.

In terms of energy, UV-rays straddle the border between ionizing and non-ionizing radiation. They have more energy than visible light, but not as much as X-rays. However, UV-rays often have enough energy to damage a cell's DNA, which means they can still cause cancer. But because they do not have enough energy to penetrate deeply into the body, their main effect is on the skin. UV-B light causes crosslinking between adjacent cytosine and thymine bases in a DNA string and leads to an abnormal covalent bond between the two bases on the same side of the DNA helix. Such abnormal bonds interfere with base-pairing during DNA replication, leading to mutations. This is called direct DNA damage. Then there is UV-A light, which can cause indirect DNA damage by creating free radicals which may trigger DNA damage.

Free radicals are atoms, molecules, or ions with unpaired electrons. With some exceptions, the presence of unpaired electrons causes radicals to be highly chemically reactive, as they tend toward losing or gaining an electron, so that all electrons in the atom or molecule will be paired. Many forms of cancer are thought to be the result of reactions between free radicals and DNA. This makes free radicals powerful mutagens, and thereby also carcinogens. Laboratory and animal research have shown, however, that antioxidants may help prevent the free-radical damage that is associated with cancer—they act like free-radical "scavengers." Antioxidants are molecules which can safely interact with free radicals and terminate the chain reaction before vital molecules such as DNA are damaged. Examples of antioxidants include beta-carotene, lycopene, resveratrol, cholesterol, vitamins C, E, and A; these come naturally with a healthy diet that includes a variety of fruits and vegetables.

Not all carcinogens are mutagens. Alcohol (ethanol) is an example of a chemical carcinogen that may not always act as a mutagen. Whereas one of its derivatives, acetaldehyde, can directly damage DNA, alcohol has other ways of causing harm—such as raising estrogen levels, acting as a solvent for other mutagens, causing lower levels of B-vitamin folic acid (folate) in the blood, and causing liver inflammation (hepatitis) or scarring (cirrhosis).

Some other substances cause cancer primarily through their physical, rather than chemical, effects on cells. Usually, such physical carcinogens must get inside the body through the inhalation of tiny pieces, and require years of exposure for cancer to develop. Asbestos belongs to his category; it is a naturally occurring mineral fiber that can cause mesothelioma, a type of lung cancer. Other substances in this category, such as wollastonite, attapulgite, glass wool, and rock wool, are believed to have similar effects. Non-fibrous particulate materials that cause cancer include powdered metallic cobalt and nickel, as well as crystalline silica (quartz, cristobalite, and tridymite).

Sometimes, even certain hormones can play a role in the development of cancer by promoting cell proliferation. Osteosarcoma, for instance, may be promoted by growth hormones. Hormones are also important agents in sex-related cancers such as cancers of the breast, endometrium, prostate, ovary, and testis, and also in thyroid cancer and bone cancer. Women who receive hormone-replacement therapy have a higher risk of developing cancers associated with those hormones (see Chapter 4). On the other hand, people who exercise far more than the average have lower levels of these hormones, and thus have a lower risk of cancer.

Fortunately, there are also so-called mismatch-repair genes, which help recognize errors in DNA before cell division takes place. DNA damage occurs more often than one might expect; it is estimated to occur in between one thousand and one million individual molecular lesions per cell per day. Many of these lesions cause structural damage to the DNA molecule and can alter or eliminate the cell's ability to transcribe the gene for which the affected DNA encodes. If the DNA does not "match" perfectly, repair genes may repair the mismatch and correct the error by using the unmodified complementary strand of the DNA as a template to recover the original information. However, if these repair genes are not working properly, errors in DNA can be transmitted to new cells. When this affects critical genes such as tumor-suppressor genes, it can increase the likelihood of tumor formation.

To summarize this section with a question: is there a connection between age and cancer? The answer is a cautious "yes." Part of the association between aging and cancer can be attributed to errors accumulated in DNA over a lifetime, and to age-related changes in the endocrine system. That is why it could be said that, if we lived long enough, sooner or later we all would get cancer. This may be another reason why there is not much hope for biological immortality in human beings.

BEHIND THE BIOLOGICAL FACTS

Once death sets in, it is all over—biologically speaking, at least. But no one knows when that is going to happen. No one knows when you are going to die—not even medical doctors. You may have a few months' warning, or you may die as suddenly as do victims of airplane disasters. The only certainty about death is that it will happen to each and every one of us some day; yet no one knows when.

Does this also mean that there is no further purpose remaining for the person who is dying or has died? This question relates to something more than leaving descendants behind to continue the family tree, or being remembered by others, or living on in achievements that others can benefit from. Instead, this question goes to a deeper level: the ultimate purpose behind the life of the very person who is dying or has died.

It is obvious that science does not acknowledge "purposes"; they are not part of the scientific vocabulary.

Scientists decided long ago that "purposes" should be removed from the scientific picture as non-measurable, non-quantifiable, non-mathematical, non-mechanical, and non-physical entities. The concept of "purpose" was taken out of astronomy by Nicolaus Copernicus, out of physics by Isaac Newton, and out of biology by Charles Darwin. Astronomers do not seek the purpose of comets or supernovas, nor do chemists search for the purpose of hydrogen bonds. Some philosophers may object that you could look at all cause-and-effect relationships as if the effect is the "purpose" of the cause, but that is another issue. In general, we could safely state that the concept of purpose plays no part in scientific explanations. The sun does not rise every morning because it "wants" to, but because it follows physical laws. Even water does not seek its own level because it "wants" to. Is that observation the end of purposes in life?

The Purpose of Life

Does the end of life mean that there are ultimately no purposes in life after all? The very fact that we can say "there is no purpose" should make us wonder. If there is no purpose in the universe at all, how were we ever to know there is no such thing as a purpose? As

C. S. Lewis put it, "if there were no light in the universe and there-fore no creatures with eyes, we would never know it was dark."

Besides, we should ask those who deny the existence of purposes what the *purpose* is of trying to prove or claim that there is no pur-pose in life. As a matter of fact, denying that there are purposes in life defeats its own claim. If it is your purpose to remove all pur-poses from life, you are also wiping out your own purpose of doing so; those whose purpose it is to eradicate all purposes from life have lost even the very purpose for doing so. That is why it is always baf-fling how some people have made it their main purpose in life to claim that there are no purposes in life.

One could even take this thought one step further: in a universe without purposes, there could not even be any man-made machines, since such machines, curiously enough, are always made for a purpose; the world of technology is per definition purpose-driven, based on purposes that designers and engineers have in mind. Therefore, we could not even ban purposes from the universe by saying the universe is just a machine that runs with clockwork precision. Using the machine metaphor to claim there is no purpose in this universe is a bit odd, to say the least.

When scientists removed "purposes" from scientific discourse, they did not make them disappear entirely; they just moved them from inside to outside the scientific domain. But that which you choose to neglect you cannot just reject. The fact that "purposes" are missing on scientific maps does not mean they do not exist at all—just think of the roads that are missing on subway maps, which do not thereby cease to exist. Something similar holds for purposes; they are not completely out of the picture, although they are out of the scientific picture.

So the question remains: can there be a purpose to life, even beyond life, after death? To be sure, death is the end of a life cycle; but to be more precise, it is the end of *biological* life. The end of the body may not be the end of the soul—in the same way as the end of the brain may not be the end of the mind (the mind being the intel-lectual part of the soul; see Chapter 5). It makes perfect sense to pose the question: why could death not be the beginning of a new and different life? True, if there is nothing else to life than molecules, death is certainly the end of life, in which all molecules disintegrate and fall apart—a point of no return. But that moment would then also be the end of our certainty that death is the end of everything in life, as all our certainties must fall apart as well—unless our certainties are not of a molecular nature and do not fall apart when our molecules fall apart. Let us put it this way again: if our beliefs were purely a matter of molecules, then our beliefs could not be true; so we do not have to believe that our beliefs are purely a matter of molecules. This may sound like a heavy philosophical statement, but it is worth pondering it in order to digest its implications.

Not only is death a necessary part of life, it could also be a necessary *stage* in life—a stage of transition into another kind of life, perhaps. What we call the last stage may very well turn out to be the next-to-last stage, when seen in a wider-than-biological context. When we came into this world, we went through a rather similar transition by leaving the protective shelter of our mother's womb (see Chapter 2). At that moment, fetal life ended, rather abruptly. It must have been a shocking, almost traumatic, experience when we were pushed out of the womb, had to go through the tunnel of the birth canal, and were forced to breathe on our own—a physical and emotional shock, for sure. At that moment, we were certainly entering a very different and unknown world. We had to trust that we could live there and that there were human hands welcoming us. We were fortunate to find out that there was life beyond fetal death. Who would choose to remain unborn after having experienced even some of the riches of life?

Something similar may be happening when we are pushed through the "birth canal of death," leaving behind the comforting world we had become so accustomed to. The transition from this life to the next stage through the process we call biological death is often painful and frightening in a similar way. If the analogies between birth and death hold true, however, we should not be so fearful; for just as this life surpassed existence within the womb, so too could the next life surpass all we have experienced here on earth—with "hands" waiting to receive us at the other end. It must be granted, though, that we have no firsthand experience of what the next life will be like—or do we? This brings us to those so-called near-death experiences.

Near-Death Experiences

A near-death experience (NDE) refers to a broad range of personal experiences associated with impending death, encompassing sensations such as detachment from the body, feelings of levitation, total serenity, security, warmth, the experience of absolute dissolution, and the presence of a bright light. These are the phenomena that are usually reported after an individual has been pronounced clinically dead or was otherwise very close to death—hence the term "near-death experience."

According to a recent Gallup poll, approximately eight million Americans claim to have had a near-death experience; however, the exact number of people who have had near-death experiences may be much higher, because those who have had such an experience may not feel comfortable discussing it with others, especially when such an experience is understood as a paranormal incident.

One of the first clinical studies of near-death experiences (NDEs) in cardiac-arrest patients was done in 2001 by Pim van Lommel, a cardiologist in the Netherlands. With his team, he studied a group of Dutch patients who had been brain-dead from cardiac arrest but were successfully revived. Of the 344 patients who were successfully resuscitated, 62 experienced "classic" NDEs, which included out-of-body experiences. Of these 62 patients, 50% reported an awareness or sense of being dead, 24% said that they had had an out-of-body experience, and 31% recalled moving through a tunnel, while 32% described meeting with deceased people.

None of those patients reported a distressing or frightening NDE. The patients remembered details of their conditions during their cardiac arrest despite being clinically dead with flat-lined brain-stem activity. Van Lommel concluded that his findings supported the theory that consciousness had continued despite lack of neuronal activity in the brain. What such experiences suggest is that the soul—and its intellectual component, the mind—can survive brain-death. If these findings are confirmed, there could be mental activities without neural activities associated with flat EEGs.

Later on, it was found that NDE subjects subsequently showed increased neural activity in the left temporal lobe. NDEs were also associated with changes in personality and outlook on life. Among these changes, one finds a greater appreciation for life, higher self-esteem, greater compassion for others, a heightened sense of purpose and self-understanding, a desire to learn, elevated spirituality, and a stronger sense of intuition. Changes may also include increased physical sensitivity as well as a diminished tolerance for light, alcohol, and drugs, as well as a feeling that the brain has been "altered" to encompass more and that one is now using the "whole brain" rather than a small part of it.

Many view the NDE as the precursor to an after-life experience, claiming that the NDE cannot be adequately explained by physiological or psychological causes, and that the phenomenon demonstrates that human consciousness can function independently of brain activity. No wonder NDE is often cited as evidence for the existence of the human soul, the afterlife, and perhaps even heaven and hell—concepts well-known from certain religious traditions. Many individuals who experience an NDE do see it as a verification of the existence of an after-life—including those with agnostic or atheist inclinations before the experience. In her memoir *To Heaven and Back: A Doctor's Extraordinary Account of Her Death, Heaven, Angels and Life Again*, spinal surgeon Mary C. Neal, M.D., explains how, in her own NDE, she was drowning in a kayak until God told her she still had other work to do.

On the other hand, not surprisingly, all kinds of alternative *biological* explanations have been suggested: oxygen-deprivation (anoxia), high carbon-monoxide levels, REM-sleep phenomena, psychedelic agents, hallucination. However, the question remains why not all people have an NDE under those conditions. Besides, further research has ruled these explanations out. A recent study by Dr. Sam Parnia suggests that NDE patients are "effectively dead," displaying none of the neural activities necessary for dreaming or hallucination. Additionally, in order to rule out the possibility that near-death experiences result from lack of oxygen, Parnia rigorously monitored the concentrations thereof in the patients' blood, and found that none of those who underwent the experiences had low levels of oxygen. He was also able to rule out claims that unusual combinations of drugs were to blame because the resuscitation procedure was the same in every case, regardless of whether they had a near-death experience or not.

Does a near-death experience change one's life? For some it does, for others it does not. However, that does not mean the experience is therefore not real. People who survive disastrous traffic accidents may react very differently to such a "very real" event. People who go through a miraculous healing from cancer, for instance, may react very differently to the healing they received. Some people learn from it, others do not. That is up to the mind to decide. When people go through suffering, or the loss of someone very dear, some feel bitter, some less so. Isn't it striking that when Jesus was nailed to the cross, he had on one side someone who chose to be *bitter* and on the other side someone who made the decision to be *better*? Free-will gives us both options.

Perhaps we may cautiously assume that near-death experiences do offer us a peek through the "birth canal" of death—some kind of window into the afterlife. Death may not be a final destination; there may be a better destination awaiting us. Arguably, an NDE is not hard evidence for this in a scientific sense; but as they say, absence of evidence does not imply evidence of absence. We should keep in mind that most neuroscientists would not allow for any non-material explanations anyway, since they are working within the framework of what could be called the "old" paradigm that equates the mind to the brain (see Chapter 3). On a more ironic note, we may see a decrease in NDE reports as the need for transplants forces some doctors to declare brain death more quickly.

A fair response to this controversy would be to not let hard-core proponents of materialistic explanations talk away anything that cannot be counted, measured, or quantified—no matter whether it is rationality, morality, purposes in life, or life after death. Let us keep in mind that there is a real problem for those who say that physical death is the only *certainty* there is. If physical "stuff" is all that counts, then all our certainties are on their way out as well. For if I am certain that everything is physical, I would have no reason to suppose that this certainty is true—and hence I would have no reason to be certain that everything is physical.

Let us face it: when you die, you leave behind "life"—your own life. If death is really and truly death, you are destroyed forever—never again to be "you," never again to think or to feel, never again to laugh or to love. But if there is something beyond biological death, then there must be another dimension of life that we may have overlooked or misunderstood—an immaterial dimension not limited by space and time. A failure to distinguish the immaterial soul, with the mind as its intellectual part, from the material body led Duncan MacDougall, an early 20th-century physician from Haverhill, Massachusetts, to measure how much mass a human body would lose when the soul departed the body upon death. He came up with a weight of 21 grams. He mistook the soul for something material.

True, if we are just biological machines, we certainly die—and that is it. But if we are more than biological machines—bodies with a mind and a soul—then biological death may not be the end. If the near-death experiences we were discussing here are real—and indications suggest they are—then there may be a larger purpose looming in life, making our lives into a purpose-driven, even beyond death. If the purposes we had in previous stages of life were real, why must the last purpose we have in life not be real? If someone asks me, "Are we alone in this universe?," my answer would be, "no, we are not!" I am not stating here that there are also other forms of life in this universe. Perhaps there are. But even if there are, we would still be alone—unless there is a God.

So after all, death may not be a final stage on life's journey—but rather another milestone, a next-to-last stage. It could very well be a milestone on the way to the very Heaven where our capacities of rationality and morality originally came from (see Chapter 4). At this point, science has reached its limits. To transcend those limits, we need to acknowledge that we know more than what science can tell us. One of the main sources we have beyond science is what God has revealed to us in the Bible and in the life of his son, Jesus Christ.

Heaven and Hell?

Hearing all these wonderful-sounding words, we also need to acknowledge that so many people die without ever having been welcomed into life, without ever having received love, comfort, or even justice. Some of us experience rejection, violence, poverty, suffering, pain, or injustice. Some of us may not have much to live for. This is a reality that calls for a Last Judgment, as described in the Bible.

The Bible considers suffering a consequence of the Fall in Paradise. True, the "thorns and thistles" may have always been there; but since the Fall they have been felt not only as painful but also as distressing, as something "evil." St. Thomas Aquinas makes a very astute remark in this context: "Some say that the animals, which are wild now and kill other animals, were not that way [in paradise ...]. But this is entirely unreasonable. The nature of animals was not changed by the sin of man." Aquinas is right; after the Fall the *world* did not change, but *we* did. Without sin, physical evils would not rankle or embitter us. Only humans take diseases and catastrophes as something that should not be, as something that seems to be acting against them personally. Only humans can get depressed. Animals may "dislike" these things; they can certainly feel pain, but that would not rankle or embitter them. They do not address pain by asking, "Why *me*?" They do not have a "me," and since animals do not know about good and bad, they cannot ask why bad things happen to good animals.

A final judgment is the answer to many questions we might have had in life. What about all those people who have experienced so little joy in their lives, or who were given the "wrong genes"? What about all those victims of genocide, gas chambers, torture chambers, wars? What about all those people who cannot be called back to life again to receive a bit more warmth and love? What about those neglected by their spouses or their parents or their children? So many people had hoped for something good but received so much evil and suffering instead. What are we to do with all these people?

Put differently, there are too many "debit" accounts that still need to be settled—not so much those little accounts that you might like to settle with your neighbors, but rather those enormous accounts that caused sorrow, tears, afflictions, and disasters for millions of people. The fact that we speak in terms of "accounts that need to be settled" implies already that our minds can go up "into the sky" to take a mental bird's-eye view of the world. So why would we not be able also to go up "into heaven" to see everything from an even higher perspective—God's point of view, if you will? That's where the notion of a "final judgment" comes from. If there were no final judgment, those accounts would remain unsettled. In a God-less world, in a world without purposes, there is no hope those issues will ever be addressed. Yet the earth is crying out for justice!

Because we are free human beings (see Chapter 4), we will be held accountable for our choices in life. Whatever happened in previous stages of life's journey has consequences for the next stage. However, there are good and there are bad choices. Evil is a matter of bad choices; and bad choices affect not only our own lives but also those of others. That is what a final judgment is about. If there is no *instant* repayment for good or bad actions and choices, there must be a *final* repayment in the genuinely final stage of life. We need and deserve to be judged, if God is also a just God: good actions are to be rewarded with Heaven, bad ones with Hell. As St. Augustine put it, God "did not will to save us *without* us." God does not judge us on our feelings and emotions, however—for those are sometimes beyond our control—but he does judge us on our free choices in life.

From this it follows rather conclusively that the ultimate consequence of human freedom is the existence of an eternal Heaven as well as an eternal Hell. Certainly no sane person wants Hell to exist; no sane person wants evil to exist, but evil does exist. If there is evil, and if there is eternity, then Hell is a possibility. Hell is just evil eternalized. Mark Twain said he did not believe in Hell but was afraid he would go there. C. S. Lewis called Hell "the greatest monument to human freedom." Good actions are rewarded with Heaven, bad ones with Hell. *The Catechism of the Catholic Church* puts it this way: "Our freedom has the power to make choices for ever, with no turning back" (CCC 1861).

But is there not God's forgiveness? Yes, but not unconditionally.

Benedict XVI put it this way: unconditional forgiveness—the abolition of Hell—would be the kind of "cheap grace" to which the German Protestant theologian Dietrich Bonhoeffer rightly objected in the face of the appalling evil encountered in Nazi Germany in his day. If God did not will to save us *without* us, then there must be salvation as well as damnation. The after-life must be a period of repayment—for the good things we have done as well as the bad things. As C.S. Lewis put it, those "who did most for the present world were just those who thought most of the next." Fortunately, says the Catholic Church, there is also something between Heaven and Hell, some kind of "middle state"—Purgatory. It is a place or state where human imperfection is corrected in the "fire of purification" before we can enter God's Heaven, where "nothing unclean shall enter" (Rev. 21:27). This runs counter to the cheap optimism that prevails nowadays in the minds of many, holding that the life of practically everybody automatically ends up in a state of bliss.

It is obvious that we have left here the domain of science and have entered the territory of religion, more precisely that of the Catholic religion. Science has *theories* to help us understand the world, but they are subject to change—so let us not make science more than what it is. Religion, on the other hand, has *truths* we try to understand; these never change—so let us not make religion less than what it is. It reveals to us truths that no science can reach.

Euthanasia

Now that we are at it, let us face the unavoidable question: what about people who choose to die on their own watch, either by suicide or euthanasia? The answer depends on who and what we are in the core of our being. If death were just a biological phenomenon, we could certainly manipulate human life and death, as we do with animals. But such a viewpoint ignores the fact that rationality and morality set us apart from the animal world. It skips over a vital question in human life: is there not more to human life than biology? What gives biologists and physicians the right to think that biology is all there is? Let us tackle that issue first.

Science, or biology for that matter, can certainly not prove that there is nothing outside science. If you still think there is nothing outside science, then you have actually taken on the ideology of *scientism*—which is a dogmatic "creed" stating that science provides the only valid way of finding truth, thus eliminating everything that cannot be counted, measured, or quantified. The ideology of scientism has us shackled in a physical, material world. However, claiming there is only physical matter necessarily implies that this very claim does not and cannot exist, because claims are essentially non-physical. So if you think that such a non-physical claim does exist, there must be more than physical matter in this universe. That is the reason why after each section treating biological facts in this book, there is a companion section that goes behind and beyond those facts.

Supporters of scientism are ideology-driven; they hold a collection of preconceived ideas that they consider unshakable. They claim, with a dogmatic certainty, that "the real world" is solely a world of quantified material entities. They pretend that all our questions have a scientific answer to be phrased in terms of particles, quantities, and equations. Their trust is exclusively in science, since they only acknowledge one territory—the territory of science. They believe there is no corner of the universe, no dimension of reality, no feature of human existence beyond its reach. In other words, they have a dogmatic belief in the omni-competence of science. They declare science to be the epitome of rationality, so that everything else must be recognized as the very quintessence of irrationality.

In fact, however, advocates of scientism are "science-freaks" who act like the drunkard who searches for his lost car-keys near the lamp post, because that is the only place he can see in the dark. That kind of science is "lamp-post" science. To best characterize this attitude, it might be helpful to borrow an image from the late psychologist Abraham Maslow: if you only have a hammer, every problem begins to look like a nail. With this in mind, we should not idolize our "scientific hammer," because not everything may be a "nail."

One of the problems of scientism is this: how could science ever prove on its own that science is the only way of finding truth? There is no experiment that could do the trick! Science cannot pull itself up by its own bootstraps—any more than an electric generator could run on its own power. So the truth of the statement that "no statements are true unless they can be proven scientifically" cannot itself be proven in a scientific way.

In essence, scientism is an immaterial and self-refuting claim about the material world—if we consider it true, then it becomes false. It is also a baseless, unscientific claim that can only be made from *outside* the scientific realm, thus grossly overstepping the boundaries of science. It steps outside science to claim that there is nothing outside science—which is not a very scientific move. It declares that everything that cannot be counted does not count. Why would such a declaration count if it cannot be counted?

Consider the following analogy: a metal detector is a perfect tool for locating metals, but there is more to this world than metals. That is exactly where scientism goes wrong: instead of letting reality determine which techniques are appropriate for which parts of real-ity, scientism lets its favorite technique dictate what is "real" in life and then declares everything else an illusion—in denial of the fact that science purchases its success at the cost of limiting its ambition. There is so much in life that is off-limits to science.

Back to euthanasia! If there is more to life than biology, then there may also be more to euthanasia than biology. If this argument is correct, we can no longer say, "it's all about biology," any more than we can say, "it's all about money," or "it's all about sex." Yet there are still people who tend to think this way. Some say that a biological decline in body and brain entitles us to end such a life-in-decline—for "it's all about biology." Others say that big savings in Medicare can be found by reducing the expense of treating people in their last, costly years of life—for "it's all about money." What this amounts to is basically a call for "death panels." Do we really want to flirt with *euthanasia* as a biological solution to all kinds of problems in life?

Euthanasia is basically a form of eugenics (see Chapter 2). Both terms start with the prefix "eu"—which means "good"—and both are euphemisms for bad practices, making it sound as if they are unequivocally good. But, we ought to ask, good for what?. Perhaps it is "good" as seen from a biological perspective, but not necessarily good from a moral perspective, let alone a religious perspective. Eugenics basically asserts that we should breed humans as we breed animals—hence, we should be able to kill them as we kill animals when we want to.

After its origin in the late 1800's, eugenics soon developed into a brutal movement which inflicted massive human-rights violations on millions of people. The "interventions" advocated and practiced by eugenicists targeted a wide range of "degenerates" or "unfits"— the poor; the blind; the mentally ill; entire "racial" groups such as Jews, blacks, and Roma ("Gypsies"); and the "dysgenic" victims of Margaret Sanger, the founder of Planned Parenthood. All of these "misfits" were deemed to be "unfit" to live according to the despotic dogma called "survival of the fittest." This in turn led to practices such as segregation, sterilization, genocide, euthanasia, pre-emptive abortions, designer babies, and in the extreme case of Nazi Germany, mass extermination. George Bernard Shaw predicted that "part of eugenic politics would finally land us in an extensive use of the lethal chamber." And death panels will be a part of it.

No matter how you look at it, these "eugenicists" have charged themselves with the grave duty to decide who is to live and who is to die—a quasi-moral stand erroneously based on biological grounds. They think that humans are merely animals—instead of rational and moral beings—and that they can be bred and killed like animals. These eugenicists are lucky themselves that they are already born; but once they have made it to the "boat," they are happy to shove other people back into the water by following their own man-made, quasi-moral rules—which are actually immoral laws, perhaps legal, yet certainly immoral. They believe that, since genes are in full control of our lives, they have the "right" to entitle themselves to be in control of those genes. Isn't that a contradiction? Isn't that something like saying that genes are in control of genes? Instead, we should keep stressing that no one has the right to claim that there are some human lives unworthy of living.

Does this verdict also hold for people who decide on their own that their lives should be terminated, with or without a doctor's intervention? It certainly seems so. Those who promote a compassionate response to the plight of people with a terminal illness may think they are compassionate; but being compassionate means first of all comforting the sick, not helping them take their own lives. Of course, no one wants people to suffer, so we should do everything possible to alleviate their pain; advances in pain management have made it possible to effectively control the pain of terminal illnesses. Therefore, we should help people with a terminal illness by alleviating pain, not by assisting in suicide; for suicide is always a tragedy. Most religious people would add to this that life is a gift from God which is not up to us to accept or reject.

Besides, there is a very slippery slope leading from ending lives in the name of compassion to ending the lives of people with non-terminal conditions, and even ending the lives of people no longer considered useful or worthwhile. If assisted suicide is a good, then why limit it only to a select few? Doctors in the Netherlands once limited euthanasia to terminally ill patients, but now also provide lethal drugs to people with chronic illnesses and disabilities, mental illnesses, and even melancholy. In Belgium, even children are now allowed to be the target. How much lower can the Low Lands sink?

Ironically enough, there has been various shifts in the arguments for euthanasia, from eugenic grounds to "mercy-killing," then to "assisted suicide," and finally to "autonomy" and "self-determination"—which means that all people should be allowed to decide for themselves when they want to die, without interference from churches, governments, or any other authority. This was probably a rhetorical and strategic shift, but it ended up undermining its own logic when it came to legalization of doctor-assisted suicide; for "legalization" requires per definition the involvement of at least the government and medical professionals—which are elements that can only hamper any personal and individual autonomy. Once assisted suicide had been legalized in the Netherlands, in the name of autonomy, there was no longer any way to argue politically for any limits on it. This opened the way for any kind of euthanasia, even in its non-voluntary and even involuntary form. Once we adopt the principle that suicide is acceptable, even sometimes good, then the fences that legislators might try to erect around it are inevitably arbitrary.

Since then, euthanasia has often been euphemistically called "doctor-assisted suicide." It sounds so reasonable, but what exactly is reasonable about self-destruction? Paradoxically, it is based on the assumption that certain people will be better served by being dead—which is a dubious premise indeed, as Cardinal Seán O'Malley rightly put it. Not only is the term "doctor-assisted suicide" confusing—for how can it be suicide if it is assisted?—but it is also misleading—the only "assistance" the patient receives from the doctor is a prescription to be filled at a pharmacy.

Therefore, a more realistic and accurate description of "doctor-assisted suicide" would be "doctor-prescribed death." In this context, one might argue that doctors should rather be guided by their centuries-old Hippocratic Oath: "I will not give a lethal drug to anyone if I am asked, nor will I advise such a plan." How could we trust a health care system in which medical doctors save some lives but end others?

Changing terminology does not change the reality it refers to. "Aid in dying" for terminally ill patients is just a misleading and seductive term for "aid in suicide." Proponents of this kind of "aid" often deliberately avoid the word "suicide" to mask reality, and they tend to use the term "terminally ill" instead. However, not only is the *diagnosis* doctors make about a terminal illness sometimes off, but very often their *prognosis* is too, at times even by a long shot. Some physicians do not seem to learn that they don't have a crystal ball. No one should make life-and-death decisions based on someone's best guess. Words like "mercy," "dignity," and "compassion" cannot alter the fact that "mercy-killing" is a form of killing—and when done to oneself, it is a form of self-destruction. The compassion we show to the dying is not earned by things they accomplished in life any more than it should be earned by the things an unborn baby might achieve. You cannot earn or forfeit your humanity; being of human descent is enough, both in living and in dying.

Those who really provide "aid in dying" at the end-stage of life are hospice workers, hospital chaplains, nurses, counselors, psychologists, and concerned relatives—but not those doctors who provide lethal drugs to their patients, to people who are usually not even their own patients. Providing lethal drugs is a disgrace to their profession and to the final stage of life's journey. We all have the moral duty to improve the quality of life, even at the end of life. Passionate doctors should end the patient's *suffering*, not the patient's *life*. When they decide otherwise, they make all those involved accomplices in a suicide—pharmacists, nurses, family members, friends, and even society itself.

To put it in a nutshell, *all* stages of life's journey need to be protected from abuse. *All* people need to be guarded against assassins, and this is so at *all* stages of life. So it seems that each one of us has the moral right to be protected, and others have the moral duty to protect that right. We ought to protect unborn babies from abortionists, born babies from eugenicists and from infanticide-supporters, children in adolescence from child-predators, adults from rapists, disaster-victims from organ-hunters, and aging adults from mercy-killers. Those are *rights* we should claim as human beings, and *duties* we owe other human beings. No one has the right to take those God-given rights away.

As discussed earlier, moral rights and moral duties go hand in hand. If there are no duties, there are no rights. When it comes to euthanasia, there is no duty to die; so there is no right to die. Once we uncouple rights from duties, new "rights" can pop up like mushrooms. They are invented and asserted on the spot, but the question of duty is utterly lost. At best they can become entitlements, enforced by a legal system, the laws of the land. But, to reiterate, legal laws are not identical to moral laws—they should be, but all too often are not. That is the reason why Martin Luther King, Jr. called an unjust (legal) law "a code that is out of harmony with the moral law." The law of the land is not always a reflection of the moral law.

Conclusion

In the stages we have gone through in this book, we have reached the end-stage of life's journey—if there is such a thing as an end-stage. In your own life, you may still have many stages ahead of you. Hopefully, this book has helped you to learn more about them, to better anticipate them, and to help others who are still in other stages of their lives—for the simple reason that whatever happens in a previous stage may have long-lasting consequences for the next stage. That is why this book is a guide from womb to tomb—from natural conception to natural completion.

But every stage is part of one long continuum. That continuum seems to be partially pre-programmed, and yet it has many unexpected turns—depending on our surroundings, our upbringing, our experiences, our thoughts and beliefs, our own expectations and dreams. This book has tried to give a biological description as to what each stage of this continuum has in store for us and raise some questions hidden behind those biological facts.

According to ancient Greek tradition, the Sphinx is said to have guarded the entrance to the Greek city of Thebes, where she would ask all passers-by the most famous riddle in history: "Which creature walks on four legs in the morning, two legs in the afternoon, and three legs in the evening?" She would strangle and devour anyone unable to answer that question. Oedipus solved the riddle by answering: man—who crawls on all fours as a baby, then walks on two feet as an adult, and finally walks with a cane in old age. Clearly, that seems to be life's biological journey.

However, steered by chemicals, genes, hormones, impulses, thoughts, desires, plans, dreams, and ideals, life unfolds in such an intricate way that we may only have touched the surface of it—two, three, or four legs. There may be so much more beneath the surface that science cannot access. If life were only a matter of molecules, we would have only one certainty in life—the certainty that death is the definitive end of life's journey. However, if that were really true, we would not even have that certainty left; for certainties do not exist in a world of molecules, as they are immaterial entities.

That is why this book took its starting point in the material world of science, but ultimately could not ignore the Great Questions of Life and Death in the immaterial world. Let us reflect on this once more: if our beliefs were purely a matter of molecules, then our beliefs could not be true; so we do not have to believe that our beliefs are purely a matter of molecules. A profound statement like this makes us always look beyond the biological side of life's journey. Of course, we may encounter some hurdles on our journey—perhaps better called challenges—but disappointments in life, perhaps even severe ones, can be the best learning moments on life's journey. Some stages in life may even seem like a road-block, but they are still part of the journey to our final destination. Each setback may open the prospect of a comeback.

Our final destination may not be biological death but something beyond it. Death may be the last biological stage; but if there is more to human life than biology, death may be more of a next-to-last stage. This we do not know with scientific certainty, however; but it is very likely, given the fact that each one of us is more than a physical speck, more than a chemical composite, more than a biological entity. And our faith tells us the rest.

Index

Index

folic acid 31, 148
follicles 6, 12–13, 88, 121
form and matter 134
formaldehyde 146
free radicals 40, 148
free will 94, 105, 111, 115–17
freedom
  as a moral right 105
  as a rational capacity 105
FSH (follicle-stimulating-
  hormone) 12–13, 88–9

gambling 111, 115
gender 63–5, 68, 72–5, 80, 92
gender identity disorder 74–5, 92
gender theory 73–4
genes 7–11, 18, 25, 37–8, 49, 62–4,
  68–72, 91–4, 97, 99–102, 104,
  109, 111, 115–16, 120–21, 135, 145–
  46, 149, 157, 162, 167
  micro-RNA 10
  oncogenes 145–46
  pseudo- 11
  regulatory 11
  tumor-suppressor 145, 149
genetic determinism 92–3
genetic testing 48–50, 52
genital herpes 31
genitalia 31, 38, 75
genomics 11
genotype 64, 70, 91
gestational age 30
gill pouches 34
gliomas 144
gonorrhea 31
growth spurt 54

Habermas, Jürgen 110
Haldane, J.B.S. 100, 130
Harvey, William 5
hCG (human chorionic

gonadotropin) 30
hearing aids 122
Heaven 17–8, 110, 154, 156–59
hedonism 119
HeLa cell line 143
Hell 154, 157–59, 165
hemoglobin 7, 20
hippocampus 123–24
Hippocratic Oath 164
hormone replacement
  therapy 90, 149
hormones 6, 8, 12–14, 32, 34, 38,
  62, 64, 70–2, 75, 87–8, 90–1, 128,
  149, 167
HRT (hormone replacement
  therapy) 90
human papilloma viruses 128
Huntington's disease 8
hydrocephalus 33
hypothalamus 87–8
hypothermia 140–41
hysterectomy 90

immorality 104
immortality 142–44, 149
inhibin-B 13
insulin 14, 19
intellect 16, 46, 57, 86–7, 95–8, 103,
  123, 125, 131–34, 137, 151, 153, 156
intelligence vs intellect 96
introns 10
in-vitro-fertilization 47, 51
irrationality 104, 160
IVF (in-vitro-fertilization) 47, 51

John Paul II (1920–2005) 27, 51

Kaposi sarcoma herpes-virus 146
Kass, Leon 41
Klinefelter syndrome 23
Koop, C. Everett 15, 52

About the Author

Gerard M. Verschuuren is a human geneticist who also earned a doctorate in the philosophy of science. He studied and worked at universities in Europe and the United States. Currently, he is semi-retired and spends most of his time as a writer, speaker, and consultant on the interface of science and religion, creation and evolution, faith and reason.

His most recent books are:

Darwin's Philosophical Legacy—The Good and the Not-So-Good (Lanham, MD: Lexington Books, 2012).
God and Evolution?—Science Meets Faith (Boston, MA: Pauline Books, 2012).
Of All That Is, Seen and Unseen—Life-Saving Answers to Life-Size Questions (Goleta, CA: Queenship Publishing, 2012).
What Makes You Tick?—A New Paradigm for Neuroscience (Antioch, CA: Solas Press, 2012).
The Destiny of the Universe—In Pursuit of the Great Unknown (St. Paul, MN: Paragon House, 2014).
It's All in the Genes!—Really? (Amazon, 2014).
Five Anti-Catholic Myths—Slavery, Crusades, Inquisition, Galileo, Holocaust (Kettering, OH: Angelico Press, 2015).

For more info see: http://en.wikipedia.org/wiki/Gerard_Verschuuren
He can be contacted at www.where-do-we-come-from.com.